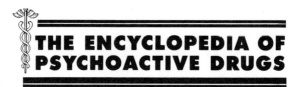

THE ENCYCLOPEDIA OF PSYCHOACTIVE DRUGS

SERIES 1

Alcohol And Alcoholism
Alcohol Customs & Rituals
Alcohol Teenage Drinking
Flowering Plants Magic in Bloom
LSD Visions or Nightmares
Marijuana Its Effects on Mind & Body
Mushrooms Psychedelic Fungi
PCP The Dangerous Angel
Heroin The Street Narcotic
Methadone Treatment for Addiction
Prescription Narcotics The Addictive Painkillers
Over-the-Counter Drugs Harmless or Hazardous?
Barbiturates Sleeping Potion or Intoxicant?

Inhalants The Toxic Fumes
Quaaludes The Quest for Oblivion
Valium The Tranquil Trap
Amphetamines Danger in the Fast Lane
Caffeine The Most Popular Stimulant
Cocaine A New Epidemic
Nicotine An Old-Fashioned Addiction
The Addictive Personality
Escape from Anxiety and Stress
Getting Help Treatments for Drug Abuse
Treating Mental Illness
Teenage Depression and Drugs

SERIES 2

Brain Function
Emotions
Mental Disturbances
Designer Drugs
Drugs of the Future
Drugs and the Brain
Nutrition and the Brain
Drugs and Disease
Drugs and Pregnancy
Drugs and Pain
Drugs and Sleep
Drugs and Perception
Drugs and Sexual Behavior
Drugs and Diet
Case Histories
Bad Trips

Substance Abuse Prevention and Cures
Using Drugs Responsibly
Drugs Through the Ages
Drugs in Civilization
Who Uses Drugs?
Drugs and the Arts
Celebrity Drug Use
Drugs and Sports
Drugs and Women
Drugs and Crime
Legalization A Debate
Drugs and the Law
Drinking, Driving, and Drugs
The Down Side of Drugs
Drug Use Around the World
The Origins and Sources of Drugs

DRUGS
&
PREGNANCY

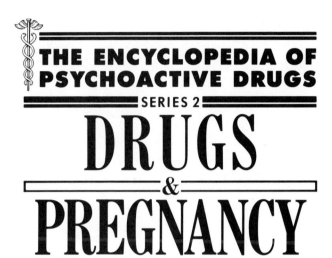

THE ENCYCLOPEDIA OF PSYCHOACTIVE DRUGS

SERIES 2

DRUGS & PREGNANCY

PATRICK YOUNG

CHELSEA HOUSE PUBLISHERS

NEW YORK • PHILADELPHIA

EDITORIAL DIRECTOR: Nancy Toff
MANAGING EDITOR: Karyn Gullen Browne
COPY CHIEF: Perry Scott King
ART DIRECTOR: Giannella Garrett
ASSISTANT ART DIRECTOR: Carol McDougall
PICTURE EDITOR: Elizabeth Terhune

Staff for DRUGS AND PREGNANCY

SENIOR EDITOR: Jane Larkin Crain
ASSOCIATE EDITOR: Paula Edelson
ASSISTANT DESIGNER: Victoria Tomaselli
COPY EDITORS: Sean Dolan, Kathleen McDermott
PRODUCTION COORDINATOR: Alma Rodriguez
PRODUCTION ASSISTANT: Karen Dreste

CREATIVE DIRECTOR: Harold Steinberg

COVER: Tchelitchew, Pavel, *Hide-and-Seek,* 1940–1942 Collection, The Museum of
Modern Art, New York. Mrs Simon Guggenheim Fund. Photograph © 1986
The Museum of Modern Art, New York.

3 5 7 9 8 6 4 2

Library of Congress Cataloging-in-Publication Data
Young, Patrick.
  Drugs & pregnancy.
  (The Encyclopedia of psychoactive drugs)
  Bibliography: p.
  Includes index.
  Summary: Examines the risks of taking drugs, both
legal and illicit, during pregnancy.
  1. Fetus—Effect of drugs on—Juvenile literature.
2. Pregnant women—Drug use—Juvenile literature.
[1. Fetus—Effect of drugs on. 2. Pregnancy.
3. Drugs. 4. Drug abuse] I. Title. II. Drugs
and pregnancy. III. Series.
RG627.6.D79Y66   1987   618.3   86-24492

ISBN 1-55546-203-0
    0-7910-0791-X (pbk.)

CONTENTS

Foreword...9
Introduction 13
Author's Preface.. 19
1 Pregnancy 23
2 Drugs and the Body....................................... 33
3 Alcohol.. 43
4 Smoking... 53
5 Drugs of Abuse 63
6 Medications 75
7 Breast Feeding 85
Appendix: State Agencies.................................. 92
Further Reading... 99
Glossary 100
Picture Credits 105
Index 106

Purchased for Parent's shelf through
Guidance Dept. Drug Free Grant,

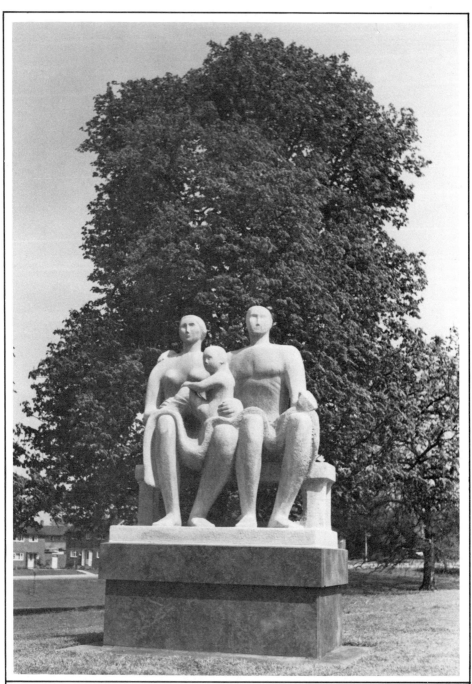

The Family Group, *as seen in this famous sculpture by Henry Moore, can become a prime victim of drug abuse, which can threaten not only parents, but their youngsters and even their unborn children.*

FOREWORD

In the Mainstream of American Life

One of the legacies of the social upheaval of the 1960s is that psychoactive drugs have become part of the mainstream of American life. Schools, homes, and communities cannot be "drug proofed." There is a demand for drugs — and the supply is plentiful. Social norms have changed and drugs are not only available—they are everywhere.

But where efforts to curtail the supply of drugs and outlaw their use have had tragically limited effects on demand, it may be that education has begun to stem the rising tide of drug abuse among young people and adults alike.

Over the past 25 years, as drugs have become an increasingly routine facet of contemporary life, a great many teenagers have adopted the notion that drug taking was somehow a right or a privilege or a necessity. They have done so, however, without understanding the consequences of drug use during the crucial years of adolescence.

The teenage years are few in the total life cycle, but critical in the maturation process. During these years adolescents face the difficult tasks of discovering their identity, clarifying their sexual roles, asserting their independence, learning to cope with authority, and searching for goals that will give their lives meaning.

Drugs rob adolescents of precious time, stamina, and health. They interrupt critical learning processes, sometimes forever. Teenagers who use drugs are likely to withdraw increasingly into themselves, to "cop out" at just the time when they most need to reach out and experience the world.

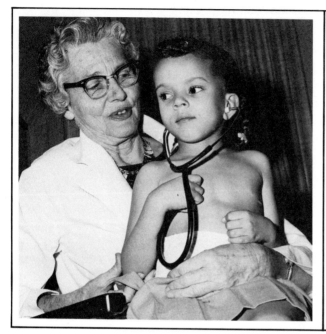

Pediatric cardiologist Helen Brooke Taussig, with a young patient in 1964. Dr. Taussig's efforts to publicize the dangers of thalidomide were largely responsible for keeping the drug, which caused deformities in the babies of the pregnant women who took it, from being marketed in the United States, thus preventing an American tragedy.

Fortunately, as a recent Gallup poll shows, young people are beginning to realize this, too. They themselves label drugs their most important problem. In the last few years, moreover, the climate of tolerance and ignorance surrounding drugs has been changing.

Adolescents as well as adults are becoming aware of mounting evidence that every race, ethnic group, and class is vulnerable to drug dependency.

Recent publicity about the cost and failure of drug rehabilitation efforts; dangerous drug use among pilots, air traffic controllers, star athletes, and Hollywood celebrities; and drug-related accidents, suicides, and violent crime have focused the public's attention on the need to wage an all-out war on drug abuse before it seriously undermines the fabric of society itself.

The anti-drug message is getting stronger and there is evidence that the message is beginning to get through to adults and teenagers alike.

The Enyclopedia of Psychoactive Drugs hopes to play a part in the national campaign now underway to educate young people about drugs. Series 1 provides clear and comprehensive discussions of common psychoactive substances, outlines their psychological and physiological effects on the mind and body, explains how they "hook" the user, and separates fact from myth in the complex issue of drug abuse.

Whereas Series 1 focuses on specific drugs, such as nicotine or cocaine, Series 2 confronts a broad range of both social and physiological phenomena. Each volume addresses the ramifications of drug use and abuse on some aspect of human experience: social, familial, cultural, historical, and physical. Separate volumes explore questions about the effects of drugs on brain chemistry and unborn children; the use and abuse of painkillers; the relationship between drugs and sexual behavior, sports, and the arts; drugs and disease; the role of drugs in history and the sophisticated drugs now being developed in the laboratory that will profoundly change the future.

Each book in the series is fully illustrated and is tailored to the needs and interests of young readers. The more adolescents know about drugs and their role in society, the less likely they are to misuse them.

Joann Rodgers
Senior Editorial Consultant

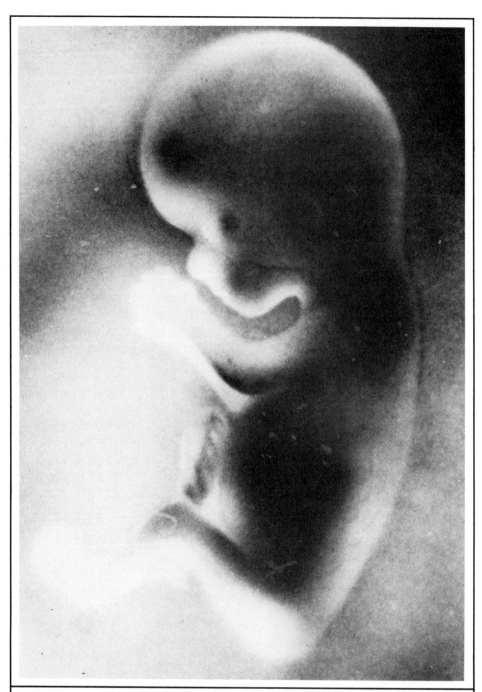

From a single fertilized cell grows a baby whose body contains several hundred billion cells at birth. At three months the major organs and circulatory system of the unborn child have already been laid down.

INTRODUCTION

The Gift of Wizardry
Use and Abuse

JACK H. MENDELSON, M.D.
NANCY K. MELLO, PH.D.

Alcohol and Drug Abuse Research Center
Harvard Medical School—McLean Hospital

Dorothy to the Wizard:

"I think you are a very bad man," said Dorothy.
"Oh no, my dear; I'm really a very good man; but I'm a very bad Wizard."

—from THE WIZARD OF OZ

 M an is endowed with the gift of wizardry, a talent for discovery and invention. The discovery and invention of substances that change the way we feel and behave are among man's special accomplishments, and, like so many other products of our wizardry, these substances have the capacity to harm as well as to help. Psychoactive drugs can cause profound changes in the chemistry of the brain and other vital organs, and although their legitimate use can relieve pain and cure disease, their abuse leads in a tragic number of cases to destruction.

Consider alcohol — available to all and yet regarded with intense ambivalence from biblical times to the present day. The use of alcoholic beverages dates back to our earliest ancestors. Alcohol use and misuse became associated with the worship of gods and demons. One of the most powerful Greek gods was Dionysus, lord of fruitfulness and god of wine. The Romans adopted Dionysus but changed his name to Bacchus. Festivals and holidays associated with Bacchus celebrated the harvest and the origins of life. Time has blurred the images of the Bacchanalian festival, but the theme of drunkenness as a major part of celebration has survived the pagan gods and remains a familiar part of modern society. The term "Bacchanalian Festival" conveys a more appealing image than "drunken orgy" or "pot party," but whatever the label, drinking alcohol is a form of drug use that results in addiction for millions.

The fact that many millions of other people can use alcohol in moderation does not mitigate the toll this drug takes on society as a whole. According to reliable estimates, one out of every ten Americans develops a serious alcohol-related problem sometime in his or her lifetime. In addition, automobile accidents caused by drunken drivers claim the lives of tens of thousands every year. Many of the victims are gifted young people, just starting out in adult life. Hospital emergency rooms abound with patients seeking help for alcohol-related injuries.

Who is to blame? Can we blame the many manufacturers who produce such an amazing variety of alcoholic beverages? Should we blame the educators who fail to explain the perils of intoxication, or so exaggerate the dangers of drinking that no one could possibly believe them? Are friends to blame — those peers who urge others to "drink more and faster," or the macho types who stress the importance of being able to "hold your liquor"? Casting blame, however, is hardly constructive, and pointing the finger is a fruitless way to deal with the problem. Alcoholism and drug abuse have few culprits but many victims. Accountability begins with each of us, every time we choose to use or misuse an intoxicating substance.

It is ironic that some of man's earliest medicines, derived from natural plant products, are used today to poison and to intoxicate. Relief from pain and suffering is one of society's many continuing goals. Over 3,000 years ago, the Therapeutic Papyrus of Thebes, one of our earliest written records, gave instructions for the use of opium in the treatment of pain. Opium, in the form of its major derivative, morphine, and similar compounds, such as heroin, have also been used by many to induce changes in mood and feeling. Another example of man's misuse of a natural substance is the coca leaf, which for centuries was used by the Indians of Peru to reduce fatigue and hunger. Its modern derivative, cocaine, has important medical use as a local anesthetic. Unfortunately, its increasing abuse in the 1980s clearly has reached epidemic proportions.

The purpose of this series is to explore in depth the psychological and behavioral effects that psychoactive drugs have on the individual, and also, to investigate the ways in which drug use influences the legal, economic, cultural, and even moral aspects of societies. The information presented here (and in other books in this series) is based on many clinical and laboratory studies and other observations by people from diverse walks of life.

Over the centuries, novelists, poets, and dramatists have provided us with many insights into the sometimes seductive but ultimately problematic aspects of alcohol and drug use. Physicians, lawyers, biologists, psychologists, and social scientists have contributed to a better understanding of the causes and consequences of using these substances. The authors in this series have attempted to gather and condense all the latest information about drug use and abuse. They have also described the sometimes wide gaps in our knowledge and have suggested some new ways to answer many difficult questions.

One such question, for example, is how do alcohol and drug problems get started? And what is the best way to treat them when they do? Not too many years ago, alcoholics and drug abusers were regarded as evil, immoral, or both. It is now recognized that these persons suffer from very complicated diseases involving deep psychological and social problems. To understand how the disease begins and progresses, it is necessary to understand the nature of the substance, the behavior of addicts, and the characteristics of the society or culture in which they live.

Although many of the social environments we live in are very similar, some of the most subtle differences can strongly influence our thinking and behavior. Where we live, go to school and work, whom we discuss things with — all influence our opinions about drug use and misuse. Yet we also share certain commonly accepted beliefs that outweigh any differences in our attitudes. The authors in this series have tried to identify and discuss the central, most crucial issues concerning drug use and misuse.

Despite the increasing sophistication of the chemical substances we create in the laboratory, we have a long way to go in our efforts to make these powerful drugs work for us rather than against us.

The volumes in this series address a wide range of timely questions. What influence has drug use had on the arts? Why do so many of today's celebrities and star athletes use drugs, and what is being done to solve this problem? What is the relationship between drugs and crime? What is the physiological basis for the power drugs can hold over us? These are but a few of the issues explored in this far-ranging series.

Educating people about the dangers of drugs can go a long way towards minimizing the desperate consequences of substance abuse for individuals and society as a whole. Luckily, human beings have the resources to solve even the most serious problems that beset them, once they make the commitment to do so. As one keen and sensitive observer, Dr. Lewis Thomas, has said,

> There is nothing at all absurd about the human condition. We matter. It seems to me a good guess, hazarded by a good many people who have thought about it, that we may be engaged in the formation of something like a mind for the life of this planet. If this is so, we are still at the most primitive stage, still fumbling with language and thinking, but infinitely capacitated for the future. Looked at this way, it is remarkable that we've come as far as we have in so short a period, really no time at all as geologists measure time. We are the newest, youngest, and the brightest thing around.

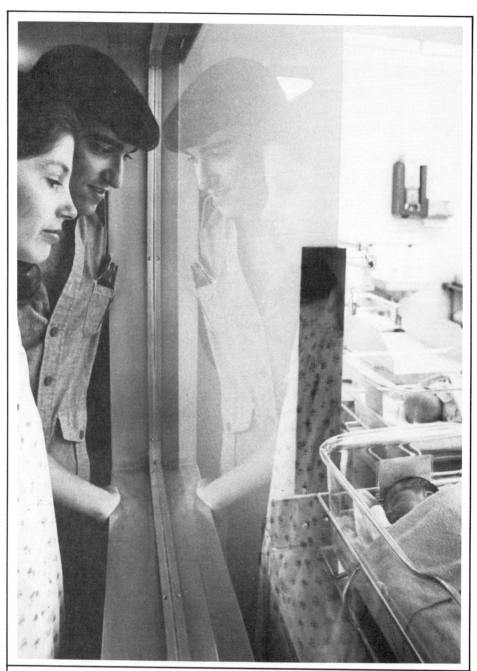

A couple looks at their newborn baby through the window of a hospital nursery. Reproduction is a complex process from beginning to end; substance abuse is dangerous to pregnant women because it can damage the fetus at any and every stage of development.

AUTHOR'S PREFACE

For many years, the unborn child was thought to be protected inside its mother's womb from any drugs or chemicals that might enter her body. But as physicians and parents alike have sadly learned, this is not true. Most drugs reach the fetus; some can do serious harm. The use of drugs — both the illicit street variety and all legal medications — during pregnancy and breast feeding is a subject of growing concern.

The United States is a well-medicated society. Early in life, Americans are vaccinated against infectious diseases and treated with antibiotics, cold remedies, pain relievers, and other medications for many ailments, some of which may be life-threatening illnesses. Many of us can count a dozen or more medications in our households. So it is not surprising that pregnant women, who usually experience a number of aches, pains, and body changes, typically take four to ten different drugs while carrying a child. Surveys show that only the elderly take more medications than expectant mothers. No doubt many of these drugs are necessary, but many more could be avoided with only mild discomfort.

The potential dangers of most drugs taken during pregnancy have not been firmly established. The same substance may be harmful or safe, depending on the circumstances. In the pages that follow, we will provide important information about the use of drugs in pregnancy and breast feeding. This volume is in no way meant as a guide to self-medication. Nor

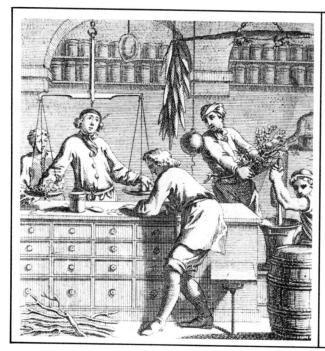

This 17th-century engraving depicts a physician measuring a dose of medicine for a patient in a primitive pharmacy. Modern pharmacology can work miracles never dreamed of two hundred years ago. Still, women cannot be too cautious when it comes to taking medication during pregnancy.

can it be considered the latest word on pregnancy and drugs. Medicine and pharmacology are rapidly changing fields. New discoveries are made, new information comes to light. Great effort has been made to provide the most recent data, but new findings are constantly becoming available. Perhaps in recent weeks new knowledge about the adverse effects on the fetus of smoking marijuana will have been revealed, or perhaps further research will have absolved a medication suspected of causing birth defects. Because our knowledge of drugs is always changing, discussing the use of medications and even illicit drugs with a doctor is a must.

The first two chapters in this book provide an explanation of what occurs during pregnancy and how drugs can help or harm the fetus. The placenta, once thought to be a protective barrier shielding the unborn fetus from harm, is a key factor. Understanding how the placenta functions, and how drugs work in the body in general, provide the backdrop for the remaining five chapters.

Chapters 3 and 4 explore the adverse effects on the unborn of two common substances that many fail to recognize as drugs — alcohol and cigarette smoke. We will look at the devastating deformities associated with heavy drinking — known as fetal alcohol syndrome — as well as other adverse effects that drinking has on the fetus. And we will discuss the physical risks and the danger of death for fetuses whose mothers smoke.

Chapter 5 examines what is known and what is not known about the effects on the fetus of illicit drug use. Women addicted to heroin and other opiates frequently give birth to babies who are themselves addicted. Other street drugs pose threats, but just how serious these threats are and how often they occur remain unanswered questions. Chapter 6 covers legal medications, both prescription and nonprescription. Some of the well-known and not-so-well-known effects of certain drugs are described, including the increased risk of bleeding in the final months of pregnancy from taking something as common and familiar as aspirin.

Finally, a baby's potential problems from drugs taken by the mother do not end at birth. Many drugs enter a woman's breast milk, and some of these can cause harm to the nursing baby. Chapter 7 explains the milk-secretion process and the drugs that are incompatible with breast feeding.

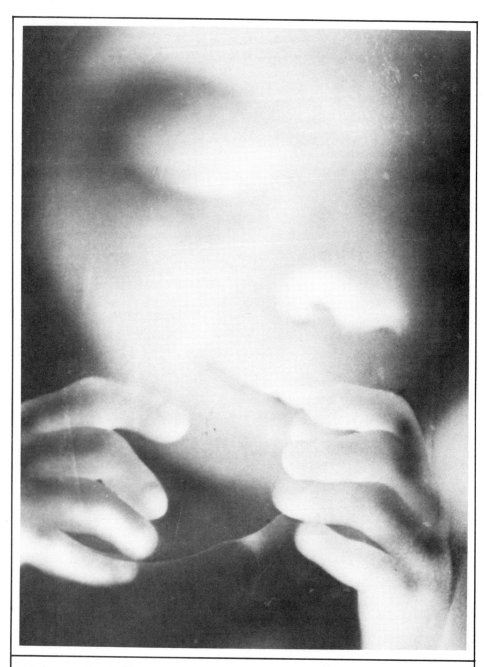

A four-and-a-half-month-old fetus. The healthy development of the fetus depends greatly on the placenta and what passes through it. This organ, formed during early pregnancy, nourishes the unborn infant but cannot protect the fetus from certain harmful substances.

CHAPTER 1

PREGNANCY

Human beings possess a marvelously diverse group of complex, vital organs — the brain, the heart, the liver, the lungs, the kidneys — each of which must function 24 hours a day, every day of our lives. Our bodies are laced by a network of blood vessels some 60,000 miles long by the time we are fully grown. Most blood vessels are so tiny that only one red blood cell at a time can pass through them. Our very existence and reproduction depends on an intricate arrangement of biochemical, nervous, hormonal, and immune systems. And finally, we possess the almost miraculous powers of thought and memory.

So it should come as no surprise that human reproduction is itself a complex process, and a unique event in the human life cycle.

During pregnancy, two genetically distinct creatures coexist, one dependent on the other for life itself. It is a time of rapid growth for the child-to-be and a period of dramatic physiological and biochemical changes for both the mother and the unborn infant. From a single fertilized cell grows a baby whose body contains several hundred billion cells at birth. Whether all these cells function as nature intended depends on many things. One very important factor is the exposure of the unborn to harmful chemicals — particularly drugs — inhaled or swallowed by the mother during pregnancy. A cigarette smoker, a heavy alcohol drinker, or a drug abuser endangers not only herself, but the child she is carrying.

Knowing what happens during pregnancy — how the unborn child is maintained and nourished within the womb — is important to understanding why drug use can be so devastating during this period in a woman's life.

Fertilization

Pregnancy begins when the body's biggest and smallest cells join together. The mature egg, produced by the woman, is the body's largest cell. A fertile woman normally releases one of these eggs each menstrual cycle. The sperm, produced by the male, is the body's tiniest cell. Several hundred million of these tadpolelike cells are released at once. Yet only one fertilizes the egg to begin the 38-week cycle of reproduction that — if all goes well — will bring another human being into the world.

A woman's body contains two ovaries, small sacs (glandular pouches) in which eggs grow and mature. Each ovary is connected to her uterus (the womb) by a tube, which is called the fallopian tube. When a mature egg is released from an ovary, it begins a journey down the fallopian tube to the uterus. If millions of sperm are released into the woman at this time, only a few hundred will survive the acid bath that awaits them in the fluids of the vagina. Many of these survivors die as they move up through the uterus and into the fallopian tubes. Some sperm take the wrong route and enter the tube that does not contain the mature egg. The few other survivors race up the correct tube. The first one to reach the egg penetrates and fertilizes it. Immediately, the egg surrounds itself with what is called the fertilization membrane, which prevents any other sperm from entering the egg.

Both a person's sex and his or her genetic makeup are determined at fertilization. Our physical characteristics — from the color of our hair and eyes to our susceptibility to certain diseases — are all determined by the hundreds of genes that make up each of the chromosomes entwined in the egg and sperm. All human cells contain 46 chromosomes arranged in pairs. The only exceptions are the egg and sperm, each of which has 23 chromosomes. At fertilization, the two sets of 23 chromosomes join to make 46. A new life is now in the making.

Immediately, the fertilized egg divides into 2 cells, a process known as cell division. These 2 cells then divide to

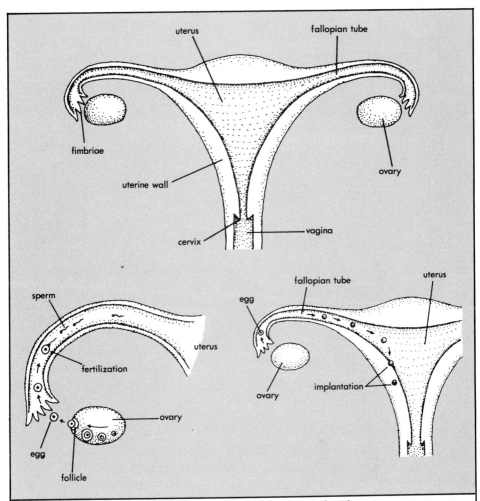

Above: The female reproductive system. Below left: The sperm penetrates the egg in the fallopian tube. Below right: Path traveled by the egg from fertilization to implantation in uterine wall.

become 4, the 4 to become 8, the 8 to become 16. This division continues as the tiny bundle of cells makes its week-long journey down the fallopian tube to the uterus. There, the cells attach themselves to the lining of the uterus. If they do not, the fertilized egg is flushed from the uterus and lost.

From two weeks to eight weeks after fertilization, the unborn child is called an embryo. From eight weeks to birth, it is called a fetus. Drugs can do damage at any time in pregnancy. But as we will see in Chapter 2, the kind of damage can be different at different stages of development.

Cell Differentiation

In the second week, the cells begin to become different, or differentiated. Some begin forming the amniotic sac, in which the unborn will live until birth. Others become the yolk sac, in which the embryo's early blood supply forms and part of which will form the beginnings of the baby's gut. Still others begin building the placenta, the organ that allows life-sustaining oxygen and nutrients to pass from the mother to her fetus. Four weeks after fertilization, the early stages of the head, neck, heart, and brain are present. By eight weeks, the nervous system and intestinal tract are evident. The heart is pumping some blood. The head is very large for the body. Arms, legs, hands, and knees are recognizable. And the placenta is functioning to support the fetus as it continues its remarkable growth and maturing.

In the remaining seven months, the fetus will grow from roughly the size of a small toe to typically 19 inches at birth. It will usually weigh about 7 pounds, perhaps as much as 10 or even 11 if delivered at full term. The brain's intricate network of nerve cells will make their proper connections. The lungs, unused in the womb, will develop and strengthen. The other organs will mature.

The Formation and Function of the Placenta

During this time, the fetus's healthy development depends greatly on the placenta and what passes through it. The placenta is a hybrid; that is, it is formed from two genetically distinct individuals — the mother and her unborn child. The outer layer develops from the mother and the inner layer from the embryo. Normally, the body's immune system recognizes genetically different tissues — such as transplanted hearts or livers — and attempts to destroy them in what is called the *rejection mechanism*. Why the body fails to reject the placenta remains an enduring medical mystery.

When fully grown, the placenta resembles a flat disk, about eight inches in diameter and one inch thick at its center. It weighs roughly one pound at birth, when it is expelled following the delivery of the baby. Normally it is attached to the upper part of the uterus. The placenta's outer side looks much like a rough sponge. It is covered with tiny, fingerlike blood vessels that burrow into the lining of the uterus to anchor the placenta in place.

A highly versatile and extraordinarily complex organ, the placenta plays many roles in ensuring the survival of the fetus. During early pregnancy, the placenta synthesizes cholesterol, fatty acids, and glycogen. It serves as a source of nutrients and energy for the embryo. It also secretes hormones vital to the growth of the fetus and the lining of the uterus. And finally, the placenta serves as a partial barrier that protects the unborn against some infections and a few drugs.

During pregnancy, the placenta plays a major role in the production of progesterone and estrogens, the so-called sex hormones that belong to a group of chemicals called steroid hormones. Estrogens perform a number of important functions. These include stimulating the growth of the uterus and the formation of new blood vessels within the uterus, and the activation of milk glands in the breasts. Progesterone prevents strong contractions that might harm the fetus. The two hormones also appear to play a role in regulating the growth of the fetus. Both the placenta and the fetus make another type of hormone — called protein hormones — and chemicals called cellular growth factors that are vital to the development to the unborn child. Much remains unknown about the exact roles of the protein hormones and how they regulate the growth factors.

William Harvey, the great 17th-century British physician known for his studies on blood circulation, was the first to recognize what is perhaps the most vital function of the placenta — it links the mother and her unborn child. Oxygen and nutrients from the mother pass through the placenta to nourish the fetus. And from the fetus, carbon dioxide and other wastes are removed through the placenta to be excreted by the mother.

Although the placenta serves to bring the bloodstreams of the mother and fetus very close to each other, the blood of the mother does not mix or come in direct contact with the blood of her offspring. The two circulation systems remain separated by a thin membrane of material called the placental membrane. The transfer of materials between the two occurs because such things as oxygen, vitamins, and fetal wastes can pass through the placental membrane.

The Umbilical Cord and Arteries

The fetus is attached to the placenta by the umbilical cord. The cord — typically one-half inch in diameter and about 22 inches long — runs from the placenta's smooth underside to the fetus's navel. It contains three large blood vessels — two arteries and a vein. These are surrounded by a soft, protective tissue called Wharton's jelly. The blood vessels inside the umbilical are actually longer than the cord itself. As a result, twisting, bending, and looping of these vessels are common.

The blood flowing in the umbilical arteries carries carbon dioxide — the gas that results when cells "burn" oxygen to provide the energy they need to function. Other fetal waste products that cross the placenta include *urea* and *uric acid* (components of urine) left over from the body's use of proteins, and *bilirubin* (the orange-colored pigment in bile, which is a secretion of the liver), which results from the normal death of red blood cells. At the placenta, the umbilical arteries pour the fetal blood into a vast network of blood vessels that carry it close to the mother's bloodstream. Only the ultra-thin placental membrane separates the two blood

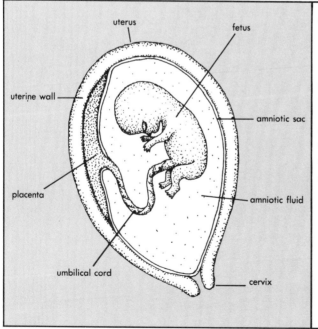

uterus

fetus

uterine wall

amniotic sac

placenta

amniotic fluid

umbilical cord

cervix

A diagram of the fetus in its mother's womb. The fetus is attached to the life-sustaining placenta by the umbilical cord. After the baby is delivered, both the umbilical cord and the placenta are expelled from the mother.

supplies. The carbon dioxide and wastes pass through the placental membrane and into the mother's blood. Her body later excretes these wastes.

Meanwhile, the mother's blood is giving up some of its life-sustaining oxygen and nutrients. Although the fetus makes breathing movements as its lungs mature, it does not actually breathe in the uterus. It depends, instead, on its mother for the oxygen it needs to survive. After the oxygen passes through the placental membrane, it enters the blood in the umbilical vein and is carried back to the fetus. There the blood is distributed, mostly to the upper body and such organs as the brain, heart, kidneys, and liver. Because the lungs are not needed for breathing at this time, they get only enough blood to help them grow. The fetal heart also works differently, since it does not have to pump great amounts of blood to the lungs until after birth.

Nourishing the Fetus

Besides oxygen, a number of other substances pass from the mother's blood through the placental membrane to nourish the fetus. These nutrients include fatty acids, proteins, amino acids (from which proteins are made), water, glucose (blood sugar), vitamins, and minerals, particularly sodium and potassium. In addition, antibodies developed by the mother to protect her against disease can cross the placenta. These provide temporary protection for the newborn infant as well, a protection that is called *passive immunity*. Unfortunately, some viruses and other organisms can also pass through the placental membrane and cause severe physical and mental defects in the fetus — or even death. These include the polio, measles, German measles, and chicken pox viruses, and the organism that causes syphilis.

Blood Flow Through the Placenta

Nothing is more important to the survival of the fetus than an adequate flow of blood through the placenta. The organ is the passageway for the substances the fetus requires for growth, and for life itself. And it is the only exit for wastes whose buildup could harm or destroy the unborn child. A reduction in the blood flow through the placenta will hinder the all-important exchange of gases — oxygen in, carbon

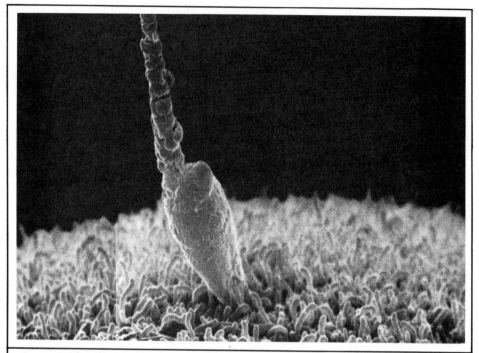

A sperm fertilizes a hamster egg. The sex of the new baby is determined immediately. All mammals share the ability not only to conceive, but also to nurture the unborn offspring within the uterus.

dioxide out — and adversely affect the quality of the nutrients that pass from mother to fetus. Thus, reducing the blood flow can result in a physically and/or mentally retarded infant, or even the loss of the fetus itself.

The placenta was long thought to be a protective shield that allowed beneficial substances to reach the fetus, but kept out potentially harmful chemicals. Indeed, the placental membrane was called the *placental barrier*. But now the placenta is regarded more as a sieve than a barrier. It allows many molecules through — and even some viruses — but blocks some very large molecules. Most licit and illicit drugs penetrate the placenta. So do many of their metabolites — the chemical byproducts that result when the body's enzymes break apart a drug so it can be cleared from the body. When drugs or their metabolites cross the placenta, the result may be helpful, harmful, or neutral.

The Thalidomide Tragedy

Although it is not the barrier it was once thought to be, recent findings show that the placenta does make enzymes that can metabolize, or alter, some drugs. Generally, drug metabolites are not as powerful or as potentially dangerous to the fetus as the original drug. But this is not always true. One notable exception is the drug thalidomide. It was widely prescribed as a treatment for morning sickness (the feeling of nausea experienced early in pregnancies) in many foreign countries — but not in the United States — during the late 1950s and early 1960s. Some 12,000 women who took thalidomide while pregnant gave birth to severely deformed children. Many of these children were born with flipperlike arms or twisted legs. In 1981, researchers at Johns Hopkins University School of Medicine discovered that it was not thalidomide itself that caused the defects, but rather a metabolite that resulted when the mother's body broke down the drug.

Harmful Substances that Cross the Placenta

The placenta also captures heavy metals — such as lead, mercury, and cadmium — that may be in the mother's bloodstream as the result of cigarette smoking or exposure to environmental pollution. Heavy metals can retard growth and cause birth defects. Trapping the heavy metals reduces the amounts of these toxins that reach the fetus. But laboratory and animal studies also indicate that cadmium, at least, can damage the placenta. This may help explain the low birth weights and other problems sometimes seen in children born to cigarette smokers.

Because it is in a state of rapid growth and development, the fetus is quite susceptible to harm from many substances that can cross the placenta. Medications are commonly used by women during pregnancy. Unfortunately, too many women also consume alcohol regularly, smoke cigarettes daily, and abuse drugs. Substances from all these pass through the placental membrane and reach the unborn child. The effects are not always apparent at birth, and are often devastating.

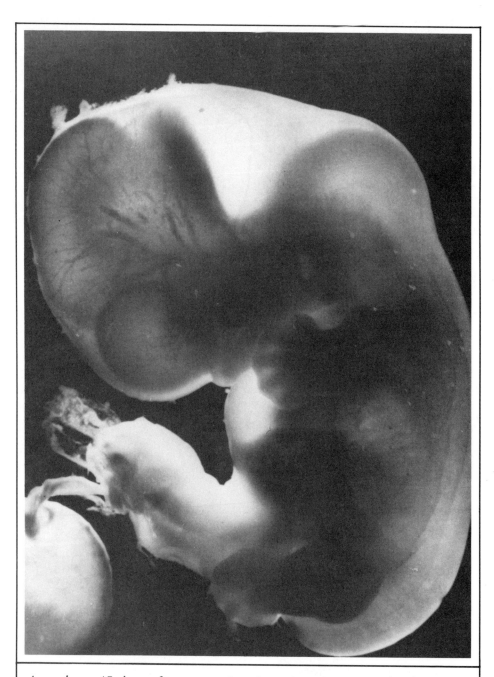

An embryo 45 days after conception; its major organs are developing and its heart is beating. During the early months of pregnancy the growing fetus is particularly vulnerable to the effects of teratogens, which are substances that are harmful to the unborn infant.

CHAPTER 2

DRUGS AND THE BODY

The human body does not discriminate when it comes to drugs. It really does not want any of them around. The body cannot distinguish between a life-saving medication and a life-threatening hallucinogen, or between a synthetic compound and a natural substance. Whether a person swallows an aspirin, gets a penicillin shot, or snorts cocaine, the body recognizes only an alien chemical molecule and goes to work to get rid of it.

By definition, a drug is a substance that changes the structure or function of a living organism. Medications are drugs whose effects on humans or animals are beneficial, or at least thought to be. Most drugs either speed up or slow down some chemical or physiological process in the body. A few medications are designed to destroy cancer cells, bacteria, viruses, or other disease-causing organisms. Obviously, all medications are drugs. But as so many drug abusers have sadly learned, not all drugs are medications.

Biotransformation

Soon after a drug is swallowed, injected, or inhaled, it enters the bloodstream and quickly spreads throughout the body. At the same time, the body is working to eliminate the ingested drug. Foreign substances in the body are either water-soluble (easily dissolved in water) or fat-soluble (readily dissolved in fat). Water-soluble drugs are removed unchanged from the blood, mostly by the two kidneys, which excrete the drugs in the urine. But fat-soluble drugs must be changed to a water-soluble form before they can be excreted. Altering a drug's chemical structure from one form to another is called *biotransformation*. It is also known as drug breakdown or drug *metabolism*. Chemicals called *enzymes* carry out the job of transforming fat-soluble drugs to water-soluble ones. Several enzyme actions that create a number of different metabolites (breakdown products) may be required before a drug is completely water-soluble. Most of this activity takes place in the liver, an organ whose prolific enzyme production makes it virtually a chemical factory in itself. However, some biotransformations occur in the intestines, lungs, and skin. Once made water-soluble, a drug can be excreted. Again, this is usually done by the kidneys, but water-soluble drugs also exit the body through sweat and through the lungs and the bile system.

Negative Complications of Biotransformation

Usually, biotransformation reduces the strength and toxicity of a drug, but not always. Although the actual effects of most drug metabolites on the body are unknown, some of these breakdown products can be even more harmful than the original substance. Remember, it was actually a metabolite and not the drug itself that caused the terrible birth defects in the children of the women who took thalidomide while they were pregnant. The body's enzymes can also convert some chemicals to cancer-causing forms. And in very high doses, the pain reliever acetaminophen (used in such products as Tylenol and Excedrin) is transformed into a metabolite that can do permanent and occasionally fatal liver damage.

The combination of two or more drugs may affect the biotransformation process. For example, carbon monoxide and lead — both of which reach the bloodstream from inhaled cigarette smoke — can slow down biotransformations by interfering with the enzymes that carry out the conversion processes. Sometimes the interaction of two drugs will increase the effect of each. For example, because both alcohol and tranquilizers depress, or slow down, the central nervous system (the brain and spinal cord), it takes less alcohol than usual to get drunk if a person is also taking tranquilizers.

During pregnancy, a woman's body handles drugs differently, and the biotransformation process becomes even more complex. The liver's ability to break down fat-soluble drugs may be slowed during pregnancy because of changes in hormones. Yet an increase in blood flow through the kidneys during pregnancy means that these organs can excrete water-soluble drugs faster.

The placenta and the fetus also break down drugs in the bodies of pregnant women. Fat-soluble drugs cross the placenta more easily than water-soluble drugs. But the latter can reach the fetus, particularly if taken in high doses. Fetal biotransformation occurs primarily in the liver. Because the fetus's enzyme systems are not fully developed, the drug-conversion process takes longer than it does in the body of

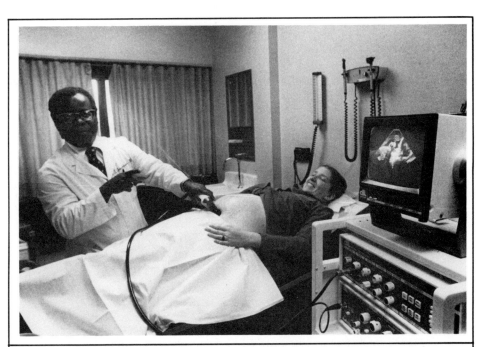

Using high-frequency sound waves, this ultrasound equipment produces a picture of the developing fetus. This technique can determine fetal position, size, some fetal damage, and a number of other features.

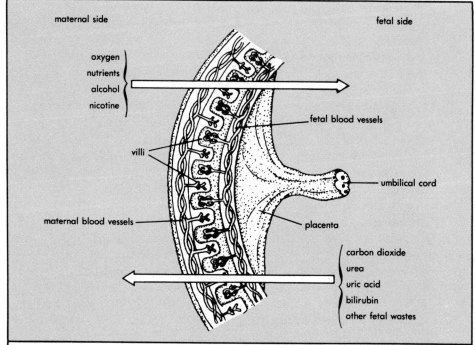

A diagram of the placental membrane highlights some of the substances that pass through the placenta between mother and child. The placenta is covered with tiny, fingerlike blood vessels.

an adult, and the drug may remain in its active form for some time. As a result, the effect of the drug on the fetus can be much stronger than it is on the mother. Moreover, it now seems likely that it is not just drug metabolites from the mother that can do harm. Some of the metabolites that result from biotransformations in the placenta and fetus may also cause birth defects or spontaneous abortion (miscarriage) of the unborn child. Clearly, the fetus can be a separate entity from its mother when it comes to processing drugs.

Drug Concentrations in the Amniotic Fluid

Drugs also may enter and concentrate in the amniotic fluid. The fetus exists inside a fluid-filled membrane called the amnion, or amniotic sac. The amniotic fluid surrounding the fetus is 98% to 99% water. It also contains a variety of salts natural to the body, carbohydrates, fats, enzymes, hormones, and pigments. Alcohol is one substance that readily passes into the amniotic fluid. It will remain surrounding the fetus in a "chemical cloud" long after the alcohol has cleared from the mother's blood. Cadmium, a toxic metal present in cigarette smoke, has been found in the amniotic fluid of women who smoke. In animals, high doses of cadmium cause birth deformities, and even low doses result in low birth weights and retarded growth.

Certainly, not all drugs are harmful during pregnancy. Sometimes drugs are necessary, even lifesaving, for either the mother or fetus. Doctors have used medications to treat unborns for such things as heart failure, low thyroid activity, and exposure to syphilis. Sometimes the benefits of medications far outweigh any possible risks, but only a physician can advise a woman adequately about drug use during pregnancy.

Drugs can adversely affect a fetus in two ways: they or their metabolites may act directly on the fetus to harm it, or they may do their damage indirectly by reducing the flow of blood through the placenta. This, in turn, reduces the supply of oxygen and nutrients to the fetus and slows the clearing of wastes — including drugs and their metabolites — from the unborn child.

Teratogens

Any substance taken during pregnancy that can cause a physical, mental, or behavioral defect in a child is called a *teratogen*. A teratogen's effects may be severe, even lethal. Or they may be so subtle, as in some learning problems, that they are barely noticeable.

Only a few of the hundreds of medications available are proven teratogens in humans. These drugs include Accutane, a prescription acne medication; tetracycline, a type of antibiotic; certain anticancer drugs; and diethylstilbestrol (DES), which was once prescribed by doctors in the belief that it prevented miscarriages. A number of other drugs are suspected teratogens, although conclusive proof of their ability to cause miscarriages or birth defects is still lacking. Indeed, few drugs are considered completely harmless.

It is, of course, unethical and immoral to perform direct tests on pregnant women to see if a drug is hazardous to their unborn children. So our knowledge of teratogens comes from less certain sources, such as studies that examine a large number of human births and analyze those in which birth defects occur in terms of any drugs the mothers involved may have taken. Other information comes from measuring the drug levels in fluid samples taken from both mother and child at birth. Yet another method involves preserving placentas expelled at birth and using them in laboratory experiments to study how and what materials cross the placenta and reach the fetus. But all of these tests have disadvantages that often leave the accuracy of their results open to question.

The administration of suspected teratogens to pregnant animals provides another source of useful but imperfect information. Unfortunately, it is difficult to apply the findings from animal studies to humans. Different species react differently to the same drugs. A medication that causes birth defects in animals may cause none in humans, and vice versa. Thalidomide was extensively tested in rats before marketing and was found to cause no birth defects. Researchers discovered years later that the reason the rats were not affected was that they do not form the metabolite that causes the terrible birth defects seen in the infants whose mothers used the drug. On the other hand, although penicillin causes birth defects in several animal species, it is regarded as one of the safer drugs that can be given to pregnant women. Animal experiments may suggest a drug will or will not be a teratogen, but they can never conclusively prove it.

McKAY DRUG Inc.
AM 1869594
301 AVE OF THE AMERICAS
Phone 255-5054 N.Y.C. 10014

No. 122957   Date 9/3/86
Henrietta Haller 293 Dahlgreen
ONE capsule 4 times a day on
   an Empty Stomach
Tetracycline 250mg
   11 18267 4/87

                    Casey
          Dr

Although tetracycline is an antibiotic with many applications, if taken during pregnancy it can slow bone growth and cause discoloration and malformation of the child's teeth.

Whether a teratogen actually causes a birth defect depends on a number of factors, including its chemical properties, the susceptibility of the fetus, the stage of pregnancy in which it is taken, the amount per dose, the number of doses, and the total length of time the fetus is exposed to the drug. By far, the most important of these is how sensitive the fetus is to the ill effects of a drug. This susceptibility is determined by the fetus's genetic makeup — that is, the specific combination of genes that it inherits from its mother and father.

Genetic Basis of Drug Reactions

Genes are made up of *deoxyribonucleic acid* (DNA) and carry the blueprints that the body uses to make all the various proteins that it needs to grow and function. People's genes determine their eye and hair color, partially set the level of their intelligence and height, and regulate how they respond to various illnesses. Certain faulty genes can cause children to be born with serious, even fatal illnesses. Usually a number of genes work together to determine how a person responds to a drug. That is why a drug may work better on some people than others, or why it may cause varying degrees of damage in different people. Most birth defects, perhaps around 60%, are thought to occur when a fetus is exposed to a teratogen to which it is susceptible. These harmful substances include not only drugs, but X rays and other forms of radiation, and some disease-causing organisms, such as the German measles (rubella) virus.

The Critical Embryonic Stage

The timing of exposure is also important. During the first two weeks after conception, when the mother may not realize she is pregnant, the fertilized egg is extremely sensitive to potentially harmful drugs. This is a time of rapid growth, when cells are dividing and multiplying. It is a time when the wrong drug will interfere with the orderly division of all the cells and cause a miscarriage.

During the embryonic stage (see Chapter 1), organ and limb formation is progressing rapidly. This is when severe physical defects are most likely to develop if the fetus is exposed to the wrong drug. Heart defects can occur that will

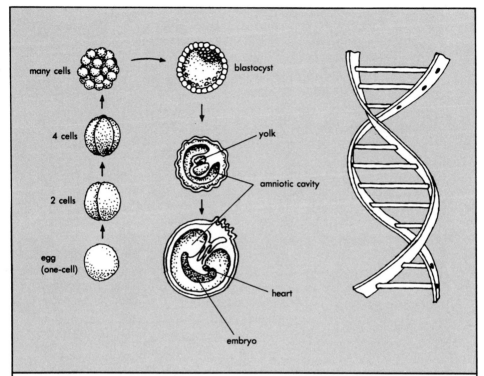

Left: Rapid cell division occurs immediately after the egg is fertilized. The blastocyst implants in the wall of the uterus and is then transformed into an embryo. Right: The DNA molecule. Among many other genetic characteristics, a fetus's susceptibility to teratogens is determined by the structure of its DNA.

require surgery after birth; damage to the brain may leave a child mentally retarded for life. The severely deformed thalidomide babies were born to mothers who took the drug during this stage of their pregnancies. Even a single dose of thalidomide taken between the 20th and 35th day after conception produced severe birth defects.

The organs are largely formed by the end of the eighth week, although considerable growth and development are still to come. The placenta is functioning, bringing about the exchanges between the blood supplies of the mother and the fetus. At this point, there is less chance that obvious physical defects will occur. But fetal growth can still be severely retarded. Subtle damage can be done to the brain that will affect the child's intelligence and ability to learn. And as doctors have learned from the drug diethylstilbestrol (DES), the teratogenic effects of a drug may not appear until years after a child is born.

DES is a synthetic form of the estrogen hormones. (A hormone is a product of living cells that is carried by the bloodstream to other cells, which it stimulates by chemical action.) DES was widely prescribed to prevent miscarriages in pregnant women for nearly 30 years, beginning in the early 1940s. But in 1971 researchers discovered that the daughters of women who took DES while pregnant had an increased risk of developing a rare form of vaginal and cervical cancer. Later, it was found that daughters of DES mothers also had an increased risk of *ectopic* pregnancies (occurring in a fallopian tube rather than in the uterus), stillbirths, and premature deliveries. There are some reports that the sons of DES mothers may be at increased risk of reproductive system abnormalities and infertility. But the question of what problems DES exposure in the uterus has created for males remains unresolved.

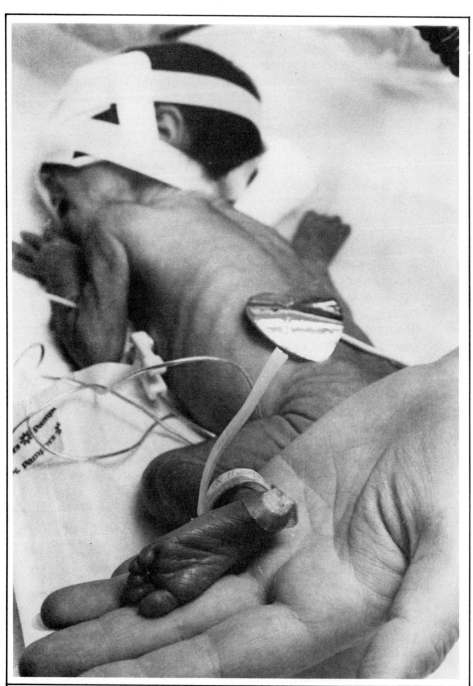

A nurse holds the tiny foot of a premature baby. Heavy drinking during pregnancy can lead to low birth weight, which increases the infant's risk of suffering physical and mental defects.

CHAPTER 3

ALCOHOL

Glenda is quite short, her head is too small for the rest of her body, and her eyes are misshapen. The middle part of her face is flattened, her upper lip is woefully thin, and her jaw juts foward. Her body is twisted by *scoliosis* (curvature of the spine) and she wears a hearing aid because she is partially deaf.

Glenda's mother was an alcoholic. Glenda (not her real name) is the victim of *fetal alcohol syndrome*, a specific set of physical and mental handicaps caused by heavy drinking during pregnancy. Today, Glenda lives with the family that adopted her, and she attends special classes for the mentally retarded. She is loved and cared for, but there is nothing that can be done to correct the devastating defects caused by the alcohol her mother consumed.

Alcohol: A Dangerous Drug

Alcohol is the world's most used and abused drug. It is an accepted part of adult life in many countries, including the United States. Beer, wine, and distilled spirits (hard liquor) are often served at weddings, parties, business and government receptions, and on innumerable other occasions. For many people, a glass of wine makes an excellent meal even more rewarding. For others, a shot of whiskey over ice or a martini straight up eases the stress of a grueling day. Unfortunately, some people develop a need for alcohol that comes to control their lives, and they become alcoholics.

The specific form of alcohol in beer, wine, and distilled spirits is known chemically as ethanol or ethyl alcohol. Ethanol is a powerful drug from a group called *general central nervous system depressants*. It slows the nerve centers in the brain that control behavior and govern the workings of the heart and lungs. Acute alcohol intoxication, especially in a young person unused to drinking, can so retard the functioning of these nerve centers that death occurs.

To be sure, scientific studies now show that moderate drinking (which is usually defined as no more than 1.5 to 2 ounces of pure alcohol daily, the amount contained in three to four 12-ounce bottles of beer or 3 to 4 ounces of 100 proof whiskey) is harmless to the health of most people. Indeed, some studies show that moderate drinking may lead to a longer life for some people by reducing their chances of suffering a heart attack.

Consuming even this amount of alcohol daily, however, may increase the chances of injury or death from traffic accidents, falls, drowning, burns, or other accidents in the home or the workplace.

Tolerance and Dependence

The dangers of heavy, sustained drinking of alcoholic beverages are even greater. Alcohol abuse can lead to *tolerance* (the need for a greater amount of alcohol to get the same effect) and physical *dependence* (addiction) — two key factors of alcoholism. Heavy drinkers are at high risk of early death from cirrhosis and hepatitis — both serious liver diseases — heart problems, cancers of the throat, mouth, pancreas, and liver, and from suicide. They are also more apt to suffer nutritional deficiencies, impotency, depression, and, in extreme cases, even irreversible brain damage.

Fetal Alcohol Syndrome

Cautions on alcohol use during pregnancy go back as far as antiquity. The Bible (Judges 13:7) warns: "Behold, thou shalt conceive, and bear a son; and now drink no wine nor strong drink." Yet it was not until the 20th century — during the 1960s and 1970s — that doctors came to recognize clearly how devastating a physical and behavioral teratogen alcohol is. In 1968 French doctors reported finding a high incidence

Drinking and Pregnancy: Potential Consequences
• Fetal alcohol syndrome (FAS) is the leading cause of mental retardation
• 30–40% of FAS babies suffer heart disease
• One-third of FAS babies suffer hearing loss
• The incidence of miscarriage or stillbirth increases when a pregnant woman drinks
• 50% of children born to mothers who drink heavily suffer from FAS
• 1 out of 650 babies born in the United States and Europe suffers from FAS
• Women who both smoke and drink are four times as likely as women who do neither to have a low-birth-weight infant

Table 1

of birth defects in children of alcoholic parents. Five years later, unaware of the French work, a team of American researchers described a specific pattern of body and nervous system defects found in 11 babies born to alcoholic women who had continued to drink heavily during their pregnancies. The American researchers called this distinct pattern fetal alcohol syndrome, or FAS. And it became apparent, as studies in the United States and abroad continued, that doctors could tell that a mother was an alcoholic simply by seeing the facial features associated with FAS in her child. The diagnosis of FAS in an unborn child could be made even if nothing was known of the mother's drinking habits.

According to the National Institute on Alcohol Abuse and Alcoholism, the cluster of birth defects that define fetal alcohol syndrome includes:

1. Growth deficiency. Babies are born small and fail to catch up despite proper nutrition.

2. A particular pattern of facial malformations. These include a small head, misshapen eyes, flattened midface, a sunken bridge of the nose, and a flattened and elongated philtrum (the groove between the nose and upper lip).

3. Central nervous system (brain and spinal cord) defects, which can result in mental retardation, alcohol withdrawal symptoms at birth, a poor sucking response and sleep disturbances during early infancy, restlessness and irritability, a short attention span, and hyperactivity.

The War of Destruction *(below)*, an 1874 woodcut by Thomas Nast, dramatizes the scourge of alcoholism, which can lead to violence, the destruction of family life, and even death.

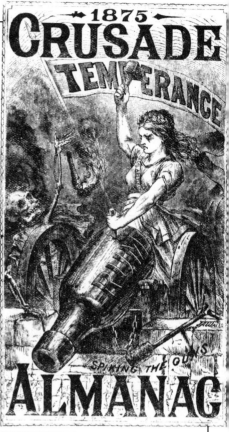

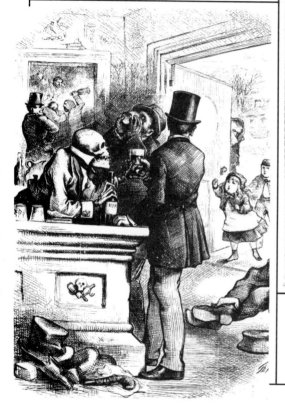

The anti-alcohol poster *(above)*, designed for the Temperance Crusade of 1875, urges total abstinence.

4. Varying degrees of malformation in the body's major organs. These may include muscle problems, defects in the bones and joints, genital defects, and kidney abnormalities.

Between 30% and 40% of FAS babies experience heart defects, ranging from mild to life-threatening. About one-third of them suffer a hearing loss and around one out of eight has a cleft palate that requires surgery. But probably the worst handicap of all is the diminished intelligence that afflicts FAS children. Fetal alcohol syndrome is regarded as the leading teratogenic cause of mental retardation.

If an alcoholic mother gives birth to one FAS child and continues to drink heavily through her next pregnancy, she is likely to give birth to an infant with even more severe defects than the first. But this is probably related to tolerance — the progressive need of the alcoholic for greater amounts of ethanol to get the same effect. Heavy drinking increases the risk that a woman will suffer a miscarriage or stillbirth. Some studies show the danger is increased somewhat even with moderate and light drinking.

Damage to the Fetus Is Dose-Related

Based on a number of animal experiments, scientists have concluded that damage to the fetus is related to the size of the dose. That is, the more the mother drinks, the worse the birth defects will be. These animal studies also indicate that susceptibility to alcohol damage varies widely among individual fetuses. And the experiments show behavioral effects occur at doses too low to cause physical deformities.

It has been estimated that as many as one-half the babies born to heavy drinkers suffer significant alcohol-caused birth defects. Although no exact figures are available, it is believed that about 1 out of every 650 babies born in the United States and Europe suffers from fetal alcohol syndrome. Moreover, for each FAS infant born, perhaps two or more are born with some of the major deformities characteristic of FAS, even though such infants may not be victimized by the full range of FAS birth defects. The National Institute on Alcohol Abuse and Alcoholism estimates that more than 40,000 babies are born in the United States each year with some form of alcohol-related birth defect.

Fetal Alcohol Effects

Doctors use a variety of terms to describe the infants injured in the uterus by alcohol who do not suffer the full fetal alcohol syndrome. These names include fetal alcohol effects (FAE) and alcohol-related birth defects. In addition to the physical damage it can do, alcohol is a behavioral teratogen as well. Both human and animal studies indicate that alcohol consumed during pregnancy can alter the fetal brain and affect infant and childhood behavior — even when there is no evidence of physical injury. Children born to moderate drinkers may show increased jitteriness, weak sucking when breast-feeding, and abnormal sleep patterns.

Minor problems with coordination and difficulty with such small motor tasks as drawing and penmanship may result from a mother's alcohol use. But the mental handicaps of fetal alcohol exposure are probably the most debilitating. Mental retardation is the most serious. But even children of normal intelligence may suffer learning disabilities and speech and language problems and have poor attention spans as the result of their mother's drinking during pregnancy. Some evidence indicates that subtle forms of these problems may occur as the result of social drinking.

Alcohol, Toxins, and the Fetus

The damage drinking does to the fetus occurs during pregnancy. So far, there is no evidence that abusing alcohol before conception results in birth defects. Alcohol quickly crosses the placenta after a pregnant woman takes a drink. The alcohol enters the fetus's bloodstream in the same concentration that exists in the mother's bloodstream. So a woman who gets drunk makes her unborn child drunk. Unfortunately, the fetus stays drunk longer. Both mother and the fetus break down alcohol in their livers so it can be excreted. But as explained in Chapter 2, the liver enzymes that do the job are not fully developed in the fetus. As a result, the fetus can take twice as long as its mother to clear alcohol from its body. Moreover, alcohol enters the amniotic fluid, which surrounds the fetus. It remains there in high concentration after alcohol has all but disappeared from the mother's blood.

Acetaldehyde, the metabolite or breakdown product of alcohol, is very toxic. It can damage cells and disrupt vital enzymes. And now there is evidence that it impairs the fetus's hormonal systems, causing some of the abnormal behavioral effects associated with alcohol. So the more acetaldehyde the fetus is exposed to, and the longer it is exposed, the more potential there is for harm.

Scientists still do not know if there is a specific stage of pregnancy during which heavy drinking is most likely to cause fetal alcohol syndrome. It may be that FAS requires a high alcohol consumption throughout pregnancy, and that the partial syndrome—the fetal alcohol effects—occurs when heavy drinking takes place only during certain stages of pregnancy. Animal research at the University of Iowa shows more damage occurs to certain parts of the brain if drinking takes place in the final months of pregnancy, rather than earlier. But many questions remain about how and when drinking does its damage to the fetus.

Polydrug Use

Women who abuse alcohol often do other things that put their unborn children at risk. Alcohol abusers tend to be heavy cigarette smokers, to abuse other drugs, and to eat nutritionally poor diets. Indeed, studies have shown that a combination of these things is more dangerous than just heavy drinking. Doctors at Boston University School of Medicine found that women who not only drink but also smoke cigarettes, use marijuana, and/or eat poorly are more likely to give birth to an FAS child than women who only abuse alcohol. In another study of 12,127 women, it was found that smokers were nearly twice as likely to give birth to low-weight babies as nonsmokers. But heavy drinkers had low-weight children almost two and one-half times more often than nondrinkers. And women who both smoked and drank were four times as likely to have a low-weight infant as those who did neither. There is no doubt, however, that alcohol by itself is the cause of FAS and lesser degrees of birth defects.

WARNING

DRINKING ALCOHOLIC BEVERAGES DURING PREGNANCY CAN CAUSE BIRTH DEFECTS

NEW YORK CITY DEPARTMENT OF HEALTH
THE CITY COUNCIL Local Law 63

A poster issued by the New York City Department of Health warns against drinking during pregnancy. This public health campaign has been gaining momentum since 1973, when researchers first discovered a correlation between certain birth defects and fetal exposure to alcohol.

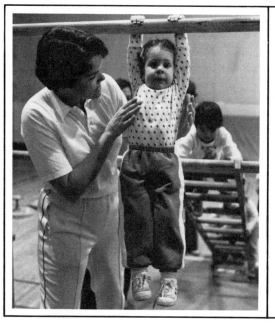

A healthy toddler participates in an exercise program designed for youngsters. Fetal alcohol exposure can cause coordination problems and developmental delays that might keep an afflicted child from engaging in normal childhood activities.

Moderation Versus Abstinence

The question remains: Just how much alcohol can a pregnant woman safely drink? Unfortunately, it is a question that cannot be answered with absolute certainty. Researchers do not know exactly how little alcohol is needed to endanger an unborn child. Any pregnant woman who drinks 3 or more ounces of pure alcohol daily — the amount contained in 6 ounces of 100 proof whiskey or six 12-ounce cans of beer — certainly risks harming her baby. A number of studies suggest there is little danger if the mother drinks less than an ounce of pure alcohol a day. Yet a study involving 31,604 live births found that even women who averaged less than one drink a day had a very slight increased risk of giving birth to a low-weight baby.

Some doctors suggest that women totally abstain from alcohol during pregnancy. Others assure their pregnant patients that an occasional drink or a glass of wine is not going to hurt them or their child. What definitely should be avoided is binge drinking—a day or two of heavy alcohol intake. There is evidence that even a single episode of heavy drinking may seriously damage an unborn child.

Some Sensible Guidelines

In 1981 the Surgeon General of the United States urged pregnant women to avoid the use of alcohol. For those who will not abstain, the federal government's Alcohol, Drug Abuse, and Mental Health Administration offers this advice concerning drinking during pregnancy:

1. Drink no more than 1 ounce of pure alcohol a day. That equals two mixed drinks containing 1 ounce of liquor each, 10 ounces of wine, or two cans of beer.

2. Two drinks a day means just that. You cannot "save up" your drinks by abstaining for three days during the week, then downing six drinks at a Saturday night party.

3. If you are accustomed to coping with tension or depression by having a few drinks, do not fill the void by using other mood-altering drugs, such as tranquilizers or antidepressants. Stop and think of other ways you might handle stress and other unpleasant feelings when they arise. Light exercise, a long walk, some relaxing music, or some kind of creative outlet can help you unwind. Meditation, writing out your feelings, or even pounding a pillow may help to vent your frustration.

4. If you find yourself seriously depressed or anxious and cannot seem to shake it off, consider getting outside help. Your doctor, area mental health agencies, or local women's centers are possible sources for counseling referrals.

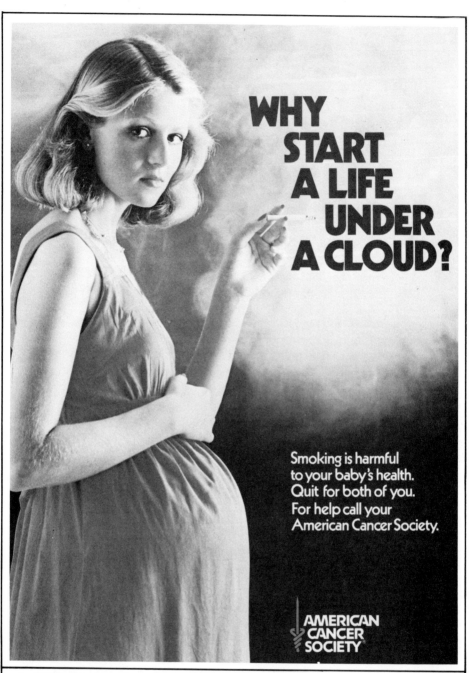

In 1977 the American Cancer Society issued this warning concerning the dangers of tobacco. Smoking during pregnancy can cause miscarriage, stillbirth, premature birth, low birth weight, respiratory ailments, behavioral disorders, or sudden infant death syndrome.

CHAPTER 4

SMOKING

SURGEON GENERAL'S WARNING:
Smoking By Pregnant Women May Result
In Fetal Injury, Premature Birth,
And Low Birthweight.

This health warning is one of four that American tobacco companies must display on their cigarette packaging on a rotating basis. It means exactly what it says. Cigarettes can harm not just the woman who smokes them, but her unborn child as well. A pregnant woman who smokes just 10 cigarettes a day increases the risk that she will bear a low-birthweight baby. One who smokes a pack or more a day significantly increases the danger that she will suffer a miscarriage or stillbirth, or that her child will die soon after birth.

The personal dangers of cigarette smoking are well documented but often ignored by millions of Americans. Cigarettes can cause heart disease, stroke, emphysema, and chronic bronchitis, as well as cancer of the lungs, throat, mouth, pancreas, and bladder. In fact, the American Cancer Society says cigarettes account for about 30% of all cancer deaths (or approximately 141,600 of the 472,000 deaths in 1986) and 83% of all lung-cancer deaths.

Cigarette smoking has declined significantly in the United States since its health dangers were first widely exposed in the now famous U.S. Surgeon General's Report of 1964. Per capita cigarette consumption — the total number of cigarettes sold per year divided by the adult population — declined from 4,141 in 1974 to 3,384 in 1985.

Disturbing Trends

Nonetheless, there are some disturbing trends. The percentage of adult smokers — both men and women — who smoke more than 25 cigarettes a day has actually increased since 1976. Cigarette use also remains popular among teenagers, and girls are more likely to smoke than boys. Moreover the U.S. Surgeon General estimates that up to 30% of women smoke during their pregnancies. Indeed, the federal government's 1980 National Natality Survey found that mothers who both drank and smoked before conception were more likely to give up alcohol while pregnant than to give up cigarettes.

Low Birth Weight and Its Consequences

Smoking during pregnancy is associated with premature birth, reduced birth weight, shorter body length, breathing difficulties at birth, behavioral and learning problems, and hyperactivity.

Many of the adverse effects of smoking during pregnancy are directly related to the number of cigarettes smoked each day. This is particularly true of low birth weight, the most frequent problem encountered in the babies of mothers who smoke while pregnant.

Low birth weight increases a child's risk of suffering physical and mental defects, illness, learning disabilities, and behavior problems. In addition, the lower the weight at birth, the lower the chances are for the infant's survival. Babies weighing less than 5.8 pounds have a significant risk of death, and those weighing 3.5 pounds or less are in even more danger.

Since 1957, more than 50 scientific studies involving hundreds of thousands of births in the United States and abroad have documented the adverse effects of a mother's smoking on her child's weight at birth. A number of factors are associated with low birth weight, including race, poverty, mother's size, nutrition, sex, and premature delivery. But cigarette smoking is independent of all these. That is, smoking by itself can lead to a low-weight baby.

According to the Institute of Medicine, a part of the National Academy of Sciences: "Smoking is one of the most important preventable determinants of low birth weight in the United States. . . . Recent studies suggest that smoking may be a significant contributing factor in 20% to 40% of low-weight infants born in the United States and Canada."

In a study of 127,000 American women who gave birth between 1979 and 1985, smokers' babies averaged 6.25 ounces less at birth than those of nonsmokers. A British study found that babies of women who smoked more than a pack a day during pregnancy are on average 11.7 ounces lighter than the children of nonsmokers. Five studies involving 113,000 births in the United States, Canada, and Wales revealed that light to moderate cigarette smokers were 50% more likely and heavy smokers more than 100% as likely as nonsmokers to have babies weighing less than 5.8 pounds. Yet a number of studies have indicated the risk of delivering a low-weight baby is quite small for women who limit their smoking to no more than 10 cigarettes a day or who quit smoking by their fourth month of pregnancy.

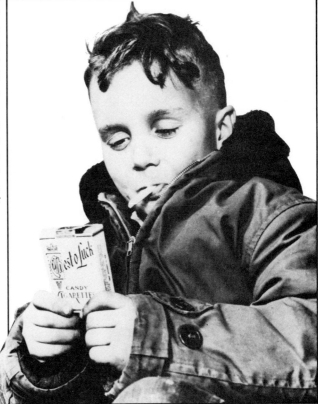

A young boy "smoking" a candy cigarette. Parents who smoke endanger their unborn offspring and can do damage to their growing children. Studies show that the children of smokers are more likely to indulge in this highly addictive habit than are the children of nonsmokers.

Low birth weights result from a slowing of a fetus's growth and development in the uterus, a condition doctors call *intrauterine growth retardation*, or IUGR. A number of different things that adversely affect the mother, the placenta, or the fetus can lead to IUGR. But they all have the same result: they interfere with the growth-sustaining flow of oxygen and nutrients to the fetus.

Smoking increases the risk of vaginal bleeding during pregnancy, which can lead to premature early delivery. Even if bleeding does not occur, smokers are still more likely than nonsmokers to deliver early. Usually, this is a matter of only a day or two. But four studies found that smokers were 36% to 47% more likely than nonsmokers to deliver two to three weeks early. Children born that prematurely face a greatly increased danger of serious complications.

Miscarriage and Stillbirth

Smoking also increases the chances of a woman suffering a miscarriage or stillbirth, or of her child dying in the first few days, weeks, or months of life. This gruesome fact has been consistently documented for almost 30 years. Studies show smokers have 30% to 70% more miscarriages than nonsmokers, and the more cigarettes smoked, the greater the danger. One study found that smoking more than a pack a day almost doubled the likelihood of a miscarriage. Stillbirths, too, increase with smoking, particularly in women whose fetuses are already at risk because certain socioeconomic factors (such as being poor or having little education) result in their receiving inadequate prenatal care. Yet a Federal Trade Commission staff study reported that 50% of American women did not know that smoking during pregnancy increased their risk of a miscarriage or stillbirth.

Sudden Infant Death Syndrome

Even if they do not have an abnormally low birth weight, the children of smokers are more likely to die in early infancy from a number of causes. Sudden infant death syndrome (SIDS), sometimes called crib death, occurs more often in the babies of smokers than those of nonsmokers. SIDS is the sudden, unexpected death of an apparently healthy child, usually between the ages of one and six months, for which

Smoking And Pregnancy: Potential Consequences
• Sudden infant death syndrome (SIDS)
• 24–68% increased chances of *abruptio placentae:* the premature separation of the placenta from the uterus wall
• 25–50% increased chances of *placenta previa:* the attachment of the placenta too low in the uterus
• 50–100% increased chances of intrauterine growth retardation (IUGR)
• Premature or low-birth-weight baby
• Slower growth in infancy and childhood
• Congenital, physical, and mental defects
• Learning disabilities
• Behavioral problems
• Respiratory diseases, such as bronchitis or pneumonia, during infant's first year

Table 2

no cause can be found. Some 6,500 to 8,000 SIDS deaths occur in the United States each year. Studies at the Hershey Medical Center in Hershey, Pennsylvania, suggest that a reduced oxygen flow to the fetus, which can occur when the mother smokes, may cause subtle brain-stem abnormalities that can lead to SIDS.

Other complications that can lead to stillbirths or early-infancy deaths include *abruptio placentae* — the premature separation of the placenta from the uterus wall. This problem is increased 24% in moderate smokers and 68% in heavy smokers. *Placenta previa*, in which the placenta is attached too low in the uterus, can lead to serious bleeding in later pregnancy. Moderate smokers have a 25% increased risk of *placenta previa*, and the danger for heavy smokers is nearly 50% greater than for nonsmokers. Both these conditions can cause a severe loss of oxygen to the unborn child — the direct cause of most smoking-related fetal deaths.

Respiratory Illnesses of Early Infancy

According to research conducted in many countries, children of smokers are especially susceptible to health ailments. A U.S. study of more than 50,000 women, called the Collaborative Perinatal Project, found that the babies of smokers tended to have lower Apgar scores than those of nonsmokers. The Apgar system is a way of rating the health of newborns. British researchers found that children of smokers suffer more bronchitis and pneumonia during their first year of life. A Finnish study reported smokers' children made more visits to doctors and were hospitalized more often and for longer periods. Several studies have shown that babies whose mothers smoke during and after their pregnancies have more illness up to age five than the children of nonsmokers do. These children are also more apt to suffer intellectual, emotional, and behavioral problems.

Hyperkinesis and Other Behavioral Disorders

Hyperactivity is more common in the children of smokers. This disorder, also called *hyperkinesis*, is a disruptive pattern of behavior that includes excitability, overactivity, poor concentration, and short attention span. A study in England and Wales found that at age 7, the children of smoking mothers tended to lag behind the children of nonsmoking women in reading skills. Concluded one University of Michigan researcher after an extensive review of the Collaborative Perinatal Project data: "Maternal smoking during pregnancy continues to show its effects long after birth, even though it is a lesser degree."

Congenital Malformations

The question of whether cigarette smoking is the direct cause of birth malformations remains controversial. Many researchers have sought the answer, but their results have been mixed. A number of studies find no evidence to link smoking during pregnancy directly with congenital malformations, while others do find an association. At least two studies have reported an increase in heart defects in the children of smokers. In 1986 a University of Kentucky researcher reported a group of specific facial deformities — including small lower jaws, small mouths, and upturned noses — among 25 children born to mothers who smoked two or more packs of cigarettes daily. And an earlier study at five large Connecticut hospitals found that smoking increased the risk that women who used tranquilizers during pregnancy would bear malformed children. Given the conflicting results so far, the possibility that smoking causes physical birth defects must not be dismissed.

Destructive Toxins in Cigarette Smoke

A great deal of evidence clearly indicts cigarettes as a fetal health hazard. Cigarette smoke contains nearly 4,000 different compounds — including some cancer-causing chemicals, cyanide, nicotine, and carbon monoxide — as well as such heavy metals as cadmium and lead.

These last two elements enter the blood whenever a cigarette smoker inhales, and they tend to concentrate in and damage the placenta. In animal studies, even low doses of cadmium result in low birth weights. In these same animal studies, at high concentrations cadmium causes miscarriages, stillbirths, and malformed offspring. Lead can interfere with the fetus's enzyme systems, and babies born to smoking moth-

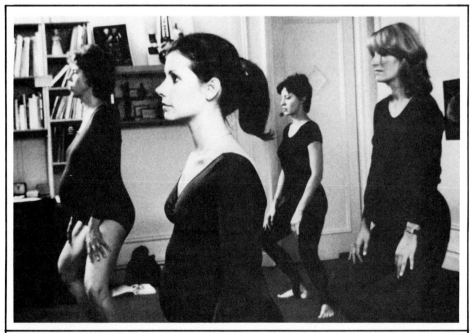

Expectant mothers exercise together. Smokers who are pregnant can do themselves and their babies a favor by substituting group support and relaxing physical activity for cigarettes.

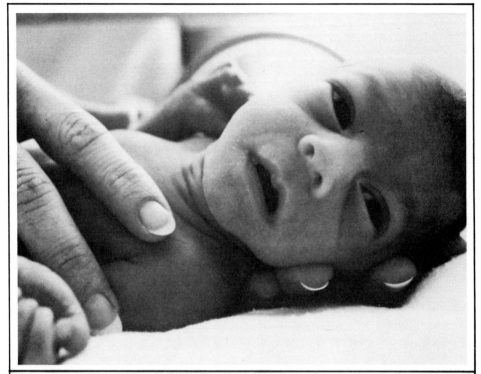

A premature baby battles for life with the help of modern hospital resources. Prematurity and low birth weight are the potentially life-threatening consequences of a number of teratogens.

ers have been found to have significantly reduced enzyme activity compared to those of nonsmokers.

Cyanide also reaches the bloodstream from inhaled cigarette smoke. It is quickly converted to thiocyanate, a substance that is normally present in the human body in minute quantities from the foods we eat. But cyanide and thiocyanate are both toxic compounds that at higher levels can reduce the ability of cells to use oxygen, interfere with the body's ability to process vitamin B_{12}, and cause damage to brain cells. Thiocyanate is a prime suspect as one cause of low-birth-weight babies among smokers.

Nicotine and carbon monoxide are the two most studied chemicals in cigarette smoke. Both cross the placenta. Nicotine causes blood vessels to narrow, including those that carry blood through the placenta. As a result, blood flow to the placenta is reduced and the organ does not function properly in supplying the unborn child's needs. Carbon monoxide is an odorless, colorless gas that kills in large doses. We all inhale some carbon monoxide, but smokers take in far more. In the blood, carbon monoxide quickly bonds to hemoglobin, the protein in red blood cells that carries oxygen. The combination is called carboxyhemoglobin. Hemoglobin's affinity for carbon monoxide is far greater than for oxygen. This means that when the two gases are present, hemoglobin will pick up carbon monoxide. The blood of smokers usually has 400% to 500% more carboxyhemoglobin than that of nonsmokers, and the level of carboxyhemoglobin in the fetus runs 10% to 20% higher than in its mother. This means less oxygen reaches the fetus. So carbon monoxide is another suspected villain in the tale of smokers' low-weight babies.

Whatever reduced health risks low-nicotine and filtered cigarettes may offer a woman do not apply to her unborn child. There is no evidence that low-tar, low-nicotine cigarettes lessen the adverse effects of smoking during pregnancy. And filtered cigarettes do not reduce the intake of carbon monoxide. The only way a woman can protect her unborn child from the hazards of smoking is to abstain from cigarettes completely during pregnancy.

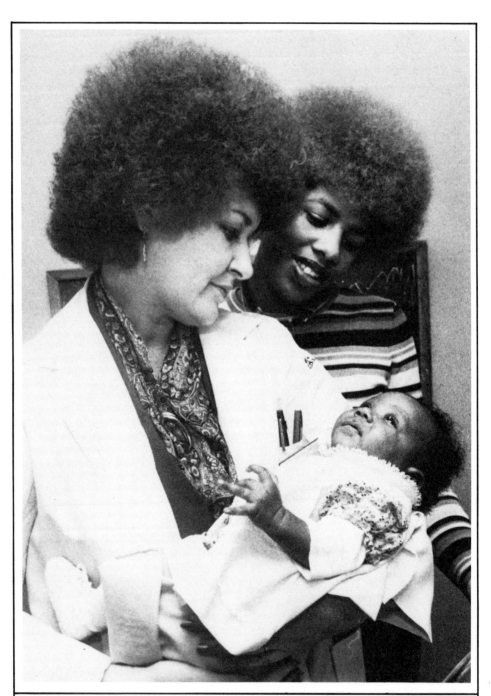

A former addict, her child, and a social worker. Up to 9,000 American children are born addicted to heroin each year. If left untreated, their withdrawal symptoms may be severe enough to kill them.

CHAPTER 5

DRUGS OF ABUSE

The use and abuse of psychoactive substances for medicinal, ritualistic, and often merely recreational purposes is as old as humankind. But the 1960s ushered in an unprecedented, virtually epidemic level of drug abuse. Beginning in that decade, millions of Americans, young and old, "turned on." Marijuana and hard-drug use increased tremendously. Since that time, drug abuse has continued at dangerous levels

Addiction Among Newborns

Tragically, the folly of some women's experiences with psychoactive drugs is visited upon their unborn or newborn children. The babies of women addicted to opium and other narcotics, for example, are usually born addicted themselves, and suffer painful withdrawal symptoms shortly after birth. The exact ill effects of other psychoactive drugs, however, from marijuana to PCP, are less well defined.

Studying the effects of illicit drugs on pregnancy is complex and difficult. Many women addicts and abusers are reluctant to participate in such studies. Moreover, the lives they lead frequently make it almost impossible to determine exactly what might have caused their birth problems. Most smoke cigarettes, drink alcohol, use more than one illicit drug, eat poor diets, live near or below the poverty level, and receive poor medical care before and after giving birth.

The best advice is to avoid all illicit drug use, particularly during pregnancy. Experience with medical drugs shows that ill effects can be difficult to pinpoint, and may be quite subtle.

Just because doctors cannot prove a street drug causes fetal harm does not mean the drug is safe. A look at what is known about the ill effects of psychoactive drug abuse on pregnancy illustrates this.

The Opiates

The use of opium — the powerful narcotic contained in the milky juice of the opium poppy — for medicinal, religious, and social purposes goes back at least 6,000 years. The ill effects of opium were also known to the ancients. Hippocrates, the Greek physician known as "The Father of Medicine," who lived from 460 to 377 B.C.E. (Before Common Era, equivalent to B.C.), warned of "uterine suffocation" in the babies of women who used the drug.

Drugs derived from opium include morphine, heroin, methadone (a synthetic opiate used to treat heroin addiction), codeine, meperidine (sold under the brand names Demerol and Mepergan), and pentazocine (Talwin). The appeal of these potentially addictive narcotics is the euphoric state they induce. The adverse effects of opiate use of a drug during pregnancy are better documented for opiates than for any other illicit drug.

Heroin is a powerful narcotic, highly addictive and almost never used medically in the United States. Some of its ill effects on newborns were well known by the late 19th century, and others were discovered as heroin addiction increased in this century. Prolonged heroin use often severely disrupts the menstrual cycle. Because they may go months without a period, it is common for heroin-dependent women who become pregnant to dismiss the signs and symptoms as due to their drug use. Some do not recognize their condition for four or five months.

In the United States, an estimated 6,000 to 9,000 infants are born each year to narcotic-dependent women. Problems for these babies can include premature birth; addiction at birth; withdrawal symptoms ranging from mild to severe; toxemia (poisonous substances in the blood); increased risk of death in early infancy; low birth weight; small body and head size; sleep, vision, and hearing problems; delays in walking; and learning disabilities. It is widely assumed that many of these result because the unborn child is repeatedly subjected to episodes of opiate withdrawal in the uterus.

The child whose mother is dependent on opium, morphine, or heroin has a 60% to 90% chance of being addicted at birth and suffering some degree of withdrawal in the first few days after birth. Unless treated, 3% to 5% of these children will die from their ordeal. Withdrawal symptoms include irritability, hyperactivity, wakefulness, tremors, twitches, jerking, swelling, diarrhea, vomiting, breathing difficulties, and sometimes convulsions. Subtle signs of some of these may remain for four to six months after birth.

Fortunately, the opiates, including methadone, do not appear to cause malformations.

Methadone is addictive, but it does not produce the euphoria that comes with opium, morphine, or heroin. It is used in treating heroin addicts to allow them to live a more stable life. Women in methadone programs generally get good

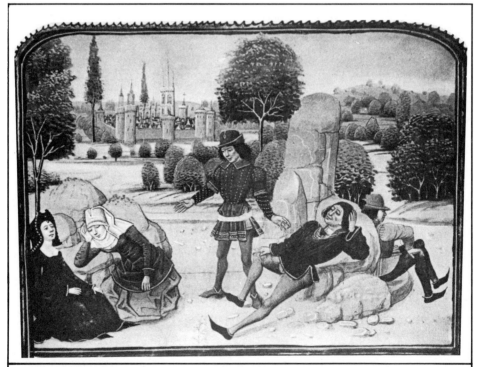

A depiction of Morpheus, Greek god of sleep, after whom the narcotic morphine was named. Mothers dependent on opium, morphine, or heroin have a 60% to 90% chance of giving birth to an addicted infant.

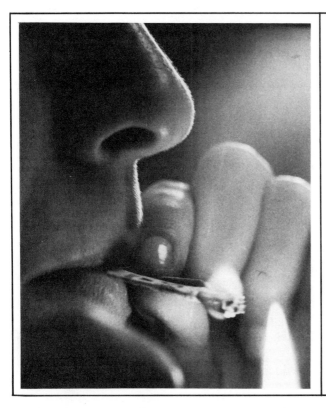

A young man smoking a marijuana cigarette. Although there is no hard evidence linking marijuana to birth defects, experts agree that until more information is available, women should avoid this drug during pregnancy.

medical care and are watched closely during pregnancy. The children of methadone-dependent mothers, although lower in birth weight than those of nonaddicted mothers, tend to be heavier than those of heroin addicts and less likely to be born prematurely. Nevertheless, about 80% are born methadone-dependent and suffer withdrawal symptoms.

Marijuana

Commonly called *pot* or *grass*, marijuana, which is the nation's most widely abused illicit drug, produces mild euphoria and sometimes sleepiness. Like cigarettes, marijuana smoke contains thousands of chemicals. The most psychoactive of these is known as delta-9-tetrahydrocannabinol.

Because of its wide use among women in their childbearing years, there has been concern about marijuana's effects during pregnancy. The drug is a potential teratogen; animal studies have shown that crude extracts of marijuana can cause brain, spinal cord, limb, and liver malformations. However, a comprehensive review of the scientific literature on marijuana by the Institute of Medicine, part of the prestigious National Academy of Sciences, failed to find absolute evidence that marijuana is a human teratogen.

"There is no evidence yet of any teratogenic effects of high frequency or consistent association with the drug," the institute's 1982 report stated. "There are isolated reports of congenital anomalies [birth defects] in the offspring of marijuana users, but there is no evidence that they occurred more often in users than in nonusers and in those cases there was coincident use of other drugs. Subtle development effects in offspring, such as nervous system abnormalities, and reductions in birth weight and height may indeed exist." The report concluded: "It may be impossible to identify a distinct role for cannabis [marijuana] in the production of subtle effects in offspring, because of the confounding influences of malnutrition, smoking, and alcohol."

Findings from a later study of 12,424 women who gave birth at Brigham and Women's Hospital in Boston are similar. The women who smoked marijuana were more likely to have premature, low-birth-weight, and malformed babies than those who did not. But when researchers took into consideration other things that might cause low birth weights, smoking marijuana was no longer a statistically significant factor. And although birth malformations were higher in marijuana-using mothers, no specific birth defects stood out as positively associated with the drug's use. Yet the findings were disturbing enough that the Boston doctors warned: "Until more information is available, women should be advised not to use marijuana during pregnancy."

Another concern has been that smoking marijuana might cause genetic damage that can adversely affect the unborn child. Some tests in animals and in human cells grown in the laboratory suggest that the tar in marijuana smoke can cause abnormal cell division and the breaking of chromosomes within cells. But a number of other studies report no evidence of such damage. "Studies suggesting that marijuana probably does not break chromosomes are fairly conclusive," the Institute of Medicine report summarizes.

In recent years, the potency of marijuana sold on the street has been increasing. Many samples seized by police are now five times stronger than those peddled in the late 1970s. No one knows yet if this increased potency poses an increased threat to the fetus.

Cocaine

Cocaine ranks second to marijuana in popularity among the nation's illicit drug users. It is an extract from leaves of the coca plant that creates euphoria and feelings of confidence and energy. Cocaine may not be physically addicting, but it can cause a craving so strong that people become psychologically dependent on the drug. Heavy users suffer hallucinations, anxiety, and paranoia.

Information on cocaine and human pregnancy is limited. There is some evidence that regular cocaine use increases the risk of miscarriages. In a study at Northwestern University Medical School, 4 of 23 pregnant cocaine users suffered abruptio placentae — a premature separation of the placenta — immediately after injecting themselves with the drug, and

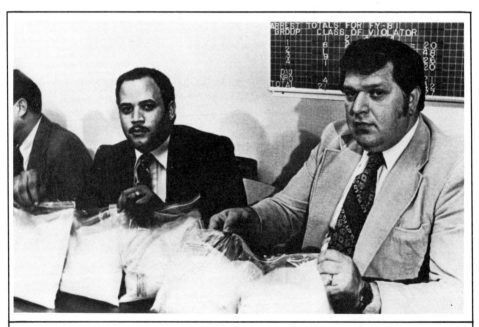

A cache of illicit cocaine. Use of this drug during pregnancy can lead to congenital malformations, miscarriages, and stillbirths.

went into early labor. In that same study, one baby died of sudden infant death syndrome. This fatality raised the question of whether fetal exposure to cocaine increases the danger of contracting SIDS.

Some animal studies have indicated that fetal exposure to cocaine causes low birth weights. But the Northwestern study found no evidence of this. Nor did it find reduction in body length or head circumference among the children born to cocaine-using mothers. Whether cocaine is a teratogen is another question. Although several animal studies report no increased danger of birth malformations, at least one found eye and skeletal defects in mice exposed to cocaine in the uterus. In the Northwestern study, one child was born with severe malformations, and the babies as a group tended to score lower on the Brazelton scale — a series of 27 reaction tests used to assess the behavior of newborns. "It is apparent from this study that cocaine exerts an influence on the outcome of pregnancy as well as on neonatal neurobehavior," the Northwestern research team concluded. "It is also possible to infer from these data that infants exposed to cocaine are at risk for a higher rate of congenital malformations and perinatal mortality."

Phencyclidine (PCP)

Phencyclidine is sold under a number of street names, most commonly *angel dust*. It is particularly popular with adolescents, the age group that is most likely to have unplanned pregnancies.

PCP was introduced in the United States in 1963 as a human anesthetic. Because of such adverse reactions as agitation, mental confusion, hallucinations, muscle rigidity, and seizures, it was soon withdrawn from human medical use. Today it is used legally only in veterinary medicine.

Drug abusers began snorting, smoking, swallowing, and injecting PCP as a hallucinogen in 1965. Many suffered extreme reactions, including bizarre and violent behavior, that quickly ended PCP's popularity with all but a few users. Then, for reasons unknown, it became popular again in the early 1970s, and its use spread. In areas where PCP is now the hard drug of choice, hospitals report that traces of PCP are found in the urine of up to 70% of the people admitted to psychiatric emergency units.

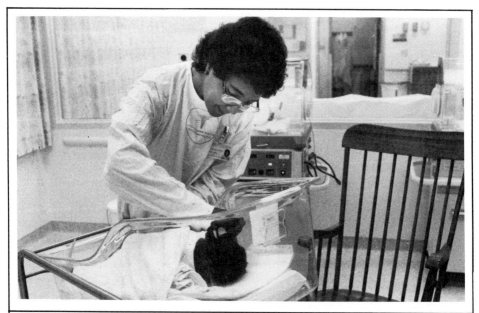

A social worker cares for the addicted child of a PCP addict. Taken during pregnancy, PCP can cause malformations at birth, and diminished reflex ability and reduced attention span in childhood.

Recent studies have shown that PCP can cross the placenta and reach the fetus. Newborns whose mothers use the drug during pregnancy may be jittery and tense and may suffer vomiting and diarrhea. They tend to have poor attention spans and decreased reflexes. There are several reports of malformed babies born to women who used PCP during pregnancy, and evidence from some animal studies suggests that the drug is a teratogen. But whether it actually causes birth defects remains unknown.

Amphetamines

Both amphetamines and barbiturates are legally prescribed medications, but they also rank high on the lists of abused drugs. Amphetamines are sometimes called *uppers* or *speed*, and barbiturates are known as *downers*.

Amphetamines were introduced in the 1930s as appetite suppressants. They cause a surge of energy, a sense of exhilaration, and wakefulness. For years they were popular with college students cramming for tests, athletes fighting fatigue, and long-distance truck drivers. More recently, their medical use has been generally limited to certain cases of obesity and a sleep disorder called narcolepsy.

Amphetamines can be swallowed or injected. When injected, the drug produces a *rush*, a sudden surge of physical energy and mental alertness. This may be followed by *crashing*, a period of depression. Long-term use can cause tolerance and psychological dependence. People who abuse amphetamines in low doses tend to be irritable and apprehensive. Long-term, high-dose use can cause brain damage, speech problems, hallucinations, paranoia, and violent behavior. High-dose users who stop suddenly suffer a long, deep depression.

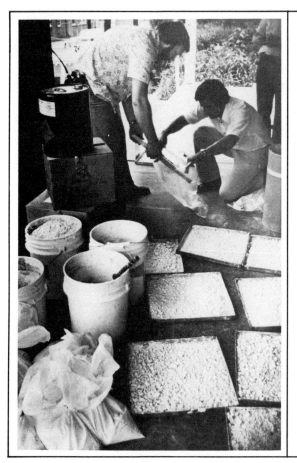

Police confiscate a doctor's illicit supply of methamphetamine. One study has found that the infants of mothers who take amphetamines during pregnancy have an increased risk of cleft lip and cleft palate.

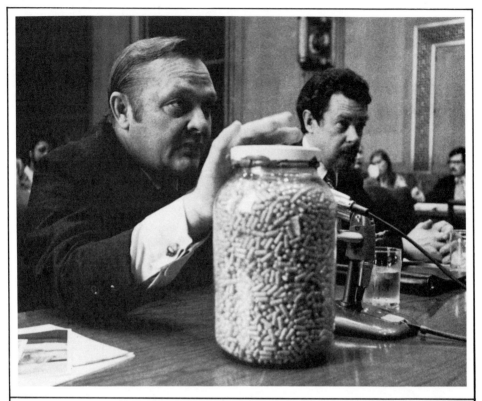

A law enforcement official displays a jar of barbiturates during a Senate subcommittee meeting. If taken during pregnancy, barbiturates can cause skin rashes, nervousness, and irritability in newborns.

There is evidence that pregnant women who use amphetamines are endangering their unborn children. Animal and human studies show that this drug increases the risk of low birth weight and premature delivery. Children born to women who abuse the drugs throughout pregnancy suffer more emotional problems. Animal studies report increased movement problems, susceptibility to disease, and early learning problems in the offspring of rats given amphetamines during pregnancy. One human study reported more infant deaths shortly before, during, or after delivery among women habituated to amphetamine who used the drug throughout pregnancy. Amphetamines do not appear to be a serious cause of birth malformations, but one human study did report an increase in cleft lip and cleft palate among infants whose mothers took amphetamines for weight control during pregnancy.

Barbiturates

Barbiturates are powerful depressants of the nerve cells in the brain and spinal cord. They are prescribed to treat anxiety, tension, insomnia, and sometimes epileptic seizures. In large doses, barbiturates are highly intoxicating. They are highly addictive and are known teratogens.

Barbiturate use during pregnancy can cause skin rashes, nervousness, and irritability in newborns. Large doses of barbiturates taken shortly before labor can cause the baby to suffer withdrawal symptoms, which include weakness, restlessness, trembling, and even convulsions. Studies with mice show barbiturates given during pregnancy can kill some developing brain cells, which results in long-term behavioral problems after birth.

Lysergic Acid Diethylamide (LSD)

Although developed in Switzerland in 1939, LSD did not make headlines until it became the drug of the "flower children" in the 1960s. Its use waned in the early 1970s as word spread about the "bad trips" it produced. Then, in the late 1970s, LSD regained some of its popularity in the drug culture.

LSD is a potent psychoactive drug. Even low doses can affect the brain and change a user's perceptions of time, distance, color, and form. These distortions of reality can last half a day and lead to anxiety or terrifying delusions. During a "bad trip," LSD users lose their sense of control, which may cause acute, terrifying panic and profound fears that they are losing their sanity. Some do suffer psychiatric problems.

Several human studies indicate that LSD use during pregnancy can cause babies to be born with deformed limbs. Two recent studies also found an increased number of eye malformations in the offspring of LSD abusers. And among 148 infants whose mothers used LSD during pregnancy, 14 suffered nervous-system defects. Interpreting all these studies is complicated by the fact that LSD users are notorious for using a variety of illicit drugs in addition to LSD itself.

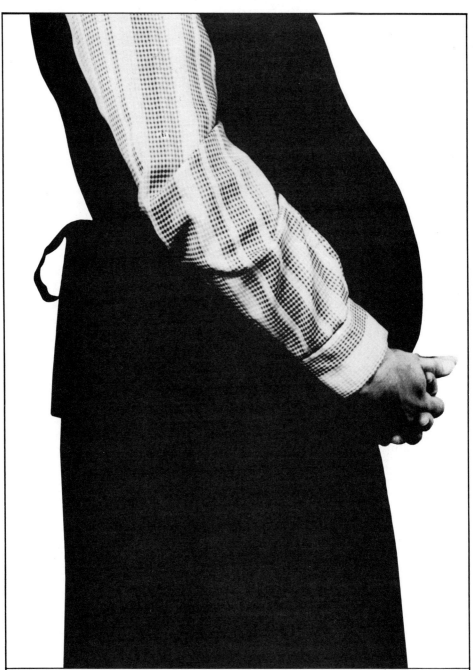

Sometimes it is necessary for a doctor to prescribe medication for a pregnant patient. Before doing so, however, the doctor must weigh the potential benefits of the drug treatment for the mother versus the possible risks to her unborn child.

CHAPTER 6

MEDICATIONS

As we have seen, the placenta was generally thought to protect the fetus against medications taken by the mother. It is now known, however, that an unborn child can be adversely affected by doses of some drugs that have minor effects on the mother. Some medications, once commonly taken during pregnancy, are no longer prescribed or are used less often. These drugs include not only thalidomide and other proven teratogens, but also diuretics (water pills), minor tranquilizers, and labor-inducing drugs.

Some Drugs Essential During Pregnancy

Some medications are clearly necessary during pregnancy. They may be needed to protect or save the life of the mother, or to prevent damage or death to the fetus. In such cases, refusal by the physician to prescribe the drug or by the woman to take it — because of misplaced anxiety about taking *any* drug during pregnancy — could cause unnecessary suffering, or worse. Drugs used to treat epilepsy and prevent blood clots, for example, pose some threat to the unborn, but ending their use might result in greater harm to the mother.

Physicians face a quandary when they consider prescribing drugs for pregnant women. Only a handful of medications have been definitely proven dangerous to the fetus. But whether most others are completely safe is really unknown. Before prescribing a drug, a physician will determine whether treatment is really necessary. If so, the next question is whether nondrug therapy will be effective. If not, then the

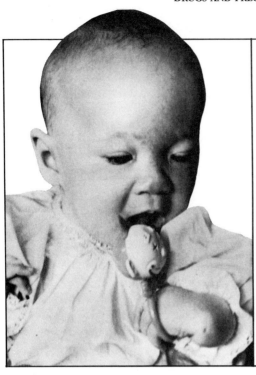

This infant was born to a woman who took thalidomide, a tranquilizer and anti-nausea pill that was widely prescribed in Europe in the late 1950s and early 1960s. Tragically, this drug caused profound birth defects in the affected babies. This child, for example, has withered arms.

physician must weigh — as best he or she can — the potential benefits of the drug treatment for the mother versus the possible risks to her unborn child.

It is important to remember that taking a drug that has a risk associated with it does not guarantee that a baby will be born deformed or injured in any way. The American Academy of Pediatrics Committee on Drugs says that a woman who takes medications for epilepsy greatly increases her risk of bearing a deformed child. Yet, the committee also notes, 9 out of 10 women who take antiepilepsy drugs give birth to normal children. A number of factors determine whether a drug will harm the fetus, such as dosage, the stage of pregnancy when the drug is administered, or the susceptibility of the fetus to that specific drug.

Proven Teratogens

We have described the horrific results for many children whose pregnant mothers took thalidomide (Chapter 1) or DES (Chapter 2). But there are other prescription drugs that can cause similar, if not quite so devastating, tragedies.

Antiacne Drugs

In 1982 isotretinoin (trade name Accutane) went on the market to treat cases of acne that did not respond to other therapies. The prescription drug was known to cause severe birth defects in animals. It has proved teratogenic in humans as well, causing fetal deaths and malformations. Women who inadvertently took the drug early in their pregnancies have given birth to babies with severe heart defects, malformed eyes and ears, small mouths, cleft palates, very small heads, and/or hydrocephaly (increased accumulation of fluid in spaces within the brain).

Accutane does its worst damage in the first few weeks of pregnancy, often before a woman knows of her condition. The drug increases by about 25 times the chance of giving birth to a deformed child. The March of Dimes Birth Defects Foundation warns that fertile women should be given a pregnancy test before the drug is prescribed, and it should be avoided throughout pregnancy.

Anticonvulsants

One out of about every 200 pregnant women suffers from epilepsy and takes medications to prevent seizures. Two of these drugs — phenytoin (Dilantin) and trimethadione (Tridione) — are proven teratogens that can cause fetal death, cleft lip, cleft palate, retarded growth, and mental retardation. The Collaborative Perinatal Project found that 11% of the women who used phenytoin during their pregnancies gave birth to babies with a specific set of defects — growth deficiency, small heads, and mental retardation — that is now called *fetal hydantoin syndrome.*

The risk of these birth defects may be reduced by switching patients to other anticonvulsant drugs. The American Academy of Pediatrics recommends that doctors discontinue the anticonvulsant medications of women who have not had a seizure for many years before they become pregnant.

Anticoagulants

Anticoagulants are drugs used to prevent or treat life-threatening blood clots that may occur after surgery, after installation of an artificial heart valve, or after a heart attack, or from a poorly functioning heart. They are "blood thinners" that interfere with the blood's clotting mechanism.

Warfarin is a commonly prescribed anticoagulant that crosses the placenta and is clearly a teratogen. (This drug is marketed under the trade names Coumadin and Panwarfin.) Its use during pregnancy, especially in the first few months, can cause fatal fetal bleeding, bone deformities, a small nose, poor vision or blindness, retarded growth, and mental retardation. Heparin (Lipo-Hepin, and others) is often used instead of warfarin during pregnancy because it does not cross the placenta. Its major drawback is that patients must learn to inject themselves with the drug.

Anticancer Drugs

Because cancer cells tend to divide more often than normal cells do, the drugs most effective against cancer work by destroying cells while the cells are in the process of dividing. It is not surprising that such drugs can be teratogens, since the cells of the fetus and placenta are constantly dividing as the fetus develops. The evidence is strongest against the drugs methotrexate and aminopterin, which belong to a group of medications known as folic acid antagonists. It is logical to expect, however, that *any* drug designed to kill cells puts the fetus at great risk. Findings from the Collaborative Perinatal Project indicate that the use of cell-killing drugs during pregnancy usually causes a miscarriage. Among those fetuses that do survive, 20% to 30% are born malformed.

Sex Hormones

DES is a synthetic form of estrogen, a major female sex hormone. Clomiphene citrate (Clomid, Serophene), an estrogen compound, can stimulate the release of mature eggs in some infertile women. But there is evidence that it can cause malformations in babies conceived after its use. Excessive androgens, the male sex hormones that create masculine characteristics in boys, can "masculinize" a female fetus as well. Androgens are found in some birth-control pills. Progesterones, a type of female sex hormone, are used alone or in combination with estrogens in oral contraceptives. Some women start to use these pills after they become pregnant but before they are aware of their condition. There is good evidence from several large studies that progesterone exposure during the first three months of pregnancy increases the unborn child's risk of limb, heart, and blood vessel defects.

The U.S. Food and Drug Administration recommends that women wait at least three months after stopping oral contraceptives before they attempt to become pregnant. A fetus conceived just after its mother discontinued her oral contraceptives may be at an increased risk of suffering birth defects.

Antibiotics

Tetracycline and streptomycin are two antibiotics that are effective against a wide variety of disease-causing bacteria. Unfortunately, they are also teratogens.

Taken during pregnancy, tetracycline (Achromycin, Robitet, others) can slow bone growth and cause the teeth of babies to be pitted and discolored when they grow in. At that time the baby's teeth are yellow, and exposure to light slowly turns them gray or brown. The pits in the enamel make the teeth more susceptible to decay. Some evidence from animal and human studies now suggests that tetracycline taken 8 to 12 weeks after conception can increase the risk of congenital cataracts, a sight-damaging clouding of the eye's lens. Streptomycin can cause a serious loss of hearing in up to 11% of the fetuses exposed to it.

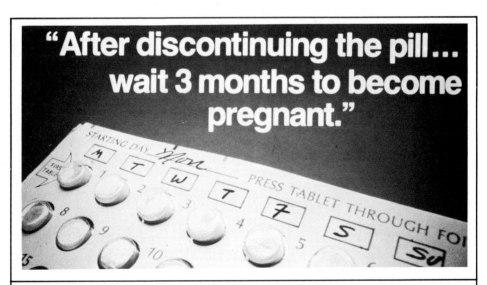

"After discontinuing the pill... wait 3 months to become pregnant."

Exposure to the sex hormones in birth control pills during pregnancy increases the fetus's risk of limb, heart, and blood vessel defects.

Lithium Carbonate

Lithium (Eskalith, Lithane, others) is the drug that revolutionized the treatment of manic-depressives, people whose moods swing between deep depression and manic excitation. Lithium is used to control the mood swings of manic-depressives, and recent evidence has shown that the drug has sharply reduced the once high suicide rate among people afflicted with this illness.

When lithium is taken during the first few months of pregnancy, though, it significantly increases an infant's risk of serious heart defects or death. The odds of premature birth and low birth weight are also significantly increased — the risk of bearing a child weighing less than 5.8 pounds at birth is almost tripled. It is believed that lithium can be used during pregnancy with considerably less danger when taken after the first three months.

Antithyroid Drugs

The thyroid gland produces hormones that regulate the body's metabolism. Sometimes this gland goes awry and produces too much of these hormones. This condition, called hyperthyroidism, throws the body's metabolism out of balance and causes such symptoms as weight loss, high blood pressure, rapid breathing, diarrhea, and muscle trembling. Women of child-bearing age are more susceptible to hyperthyroidism than are men.

The drugs methimazole and propylthiouracil (Propacil) are effective against overactive thyroids. But if given to pregnant women, they can cause drastic damage to the fetus, including goiter (an enlargement of the thyroid), hypothyroidism (low thyroid-hormone production), and cretinism, a condition resulting from the thyroid deficiency early in life that is marked by mental retardation, dwarfism, and physical malformations. Methimazole also has been associated with an ulcerlike scalp defect. Thyroid drugs are sometimes used during pregnancy when the benefit to the mother appears worth the risk. These women must be watched carefully.

Inorganic iodides have also been used to treat hyperthyroidism and can cause problems similar to methimazole and propylthiouracil. A number of asthma and bronchitis medications contain iodides, and those that do should be avoided during pregnancy.

Radiochemicals

One of medicine's "modern miracles" is the use of tiny amounts of radioactive chemicals — or radioisotopes — to diagnose a number of diseases and disorders. After it is swallowed, radioactive iodine, for example, concentrates in the thyroid, where it can be seen on an X ray. Doctors can then examine the gland for certain defects or tumors by studying where in the thyroid the radioactive material concentrates. The tiny amounts of radiation given off by radioactive iodine are harmless to adults. But if they reach the fetus, they can permanently damage the unborn child's thyroid. Other radiochemicals used in medicine can damage fetal bone or bone marrow, the soft tissue inside the bones that produces the blood cells.

Other Medications

Not only is there solid evidence to indict the specific medications discussed above as teratogens, but many more prescription drugs are suspected of causing trouble for a small percentage of babies if used during pregnancy. The antimalaria drug chloroquine (Aralen) has been associated with fetal eye damage, for example. Certain tranquilizers have been linked to heart and blood vessel defects. Dihydrotachysterol, used to treat calcium deficiency, may cause bone abnormalities. Prolonged use of the high-blood-pressure drug propranolol (Inderal) appears to increase the fetus's risk of having low blood sugar and low birth weight. Use of these or other prescription drugs may be very necessary during pregnancy, but a woman should be aware of the risks as well as the benefits of any drug she might take.

Over-the-Counter Drugs

Americans are used to going into drugstores, supermarkets, or convenience stores and buying nonprescription medications for their aches and pains. Whether it is for colds, allergies, sore throats, headaches, or any number of common ailments, we pop pills with the assumption they will make us feel better without harm. Some of these over-the-counter medications, however, pose potential and real problems for pregnant women and their unborn children. In truth, few of them are considered totally safe, because they have not been tested in pregnancy. Many liquid medications contain significant amounts of alcohol. NyQuil and Robitussin nighttime cold medications are 25% alcohol; Vicks Formula 44 cough mixture contains 10% alcohol, and CoTylenol cold medication contains 7.5%.

Even aspirin, that familiar standby of the family medicine chest, can cause problems, since it is a bloodthinner as well as a painkiller. Although the drug does not appear to be teratogenic in humans, regular use of very high doses appears to increase the risk of perinatal death. Normal doses taken in the final months of pregnancy can prolong labor and pregnancy and cause the mother to bleed heavily before and after birth. Aspirin and its chemical cousins, called salicylates, are ingredients in many over-the-counter medications that bear other names. The U.S. Food and Drug Administration recommends that women should not use aspirin products during the final three months of pregnancy without consulting a doctor.

The aspirin substitute acetaminophen, sold under such names as Datril, Tempra, and Tylenol, is now the nonprescription drug most widely used in pregnancy. Acetaminophen crosses the placenta and is metabolized by the fetus, but more slowly than by the mother. Since prolonged, heavy use of acetaminophen can cause fatal liver damage in adults, there is concern that even if lesser amounts are taken during pregnancy, the fetus may be damaged. This drug is also used in many over-the-counter medications, and a lethal fetal dose might develop if the mother takes several acetaminophen-containing products simultaneously.

Caffeine

Perhaps no commonly consumed drug has generated as much controversy in recent years about its effects on the fetus as caffeine. About 95% of pregnant women consume caffeine, a mild stimulant found in a number of soft drinks, coffee, tea, cocoa, chocolate, and many nonprescription medications. Caffeine crosses the placenta, and it has been suspected for years of causing birth defects. Findings from animal studies, however, have been conflicting, and there is no good evidence that caffeine is a teratogen in humans. Harvard University researchers who studied the pregnancies of 12,205

Aspirin is perhaps the most common over-the-counter medication, used by many pregnant women without a second thought. But in 1970 it was discovered that products containing aspirin can cause bleeding problems during labor. Brain hemorrhages in infants have also been linked to its use.

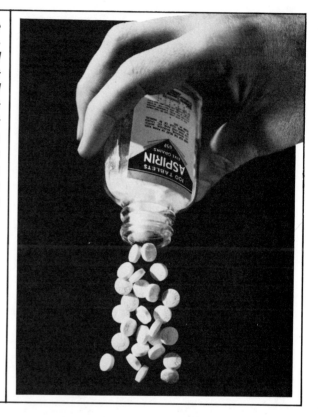

healthy, coffee-drinking women concluded, "Coffee consumption has a minimal effect, if any, on the outcome of pregnancy." Nonetheless, the Food and Drug Administration urges pregnant women to avoid caffeine or cut way back on their consumption.

No pregnant woman need panic if her doctor prescribes or recommends a drug. But every woman should realize that pregnancy is a special time when the use of medications requires extra attention. One drug carefully used may save a life; another taken carelessly may cost a life.

In the American Medical Association's *Book of Woman-Care*, authors Linda Hughey Holt, M.D., and Melva Weber offer this advice about medications during pregnancy: "Don't take anything on your own. Take only drugs that your physician prescribes. If you go to a different doctor for any reason, be sure that doctor knows that you're pregnant or trying to become pregnant."

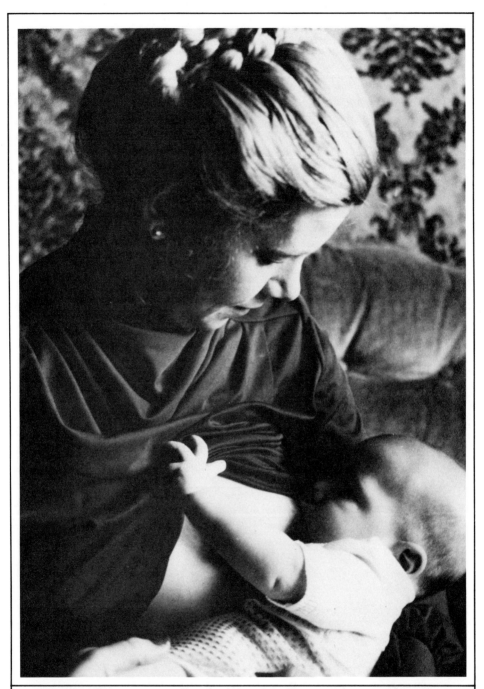

Breast milk is nutritionally ideal for the infant. Unfortunately, many unhealthy substances ingested by the mother, such as alcohol and nicotine, enter her milk supply and are transmitted to the baby.

CHAPTER 7

BREAST FEEDING

Pregnancy is, in part, a preparation for breast feeding. As the fetus develops, a woman's breasts undergo a number of important changes. The breasts first begin to grow during puberty, and they develop further during pregnancy. As the time of birth approaches, the skin appears more translucent, the veins show more prominently, and the dark area around the nipples grows even darker. Inside the breast, the milk-secreting glands and the duct system that carries the milk to the nipples prepare for the first feeding — which is sometimes the baby's first dose of a drug outside the uterus.

Almost any drug a mother takes will make it into her milk in some degree. Some of these can be damaging to a baby. Many others are safe or essentially harmless. But the ill effects — if any — of the large majority of drugs are simply unknown. Caution and consultation with her physician remain a woman's best approach to the use of drugs during the time she is breast-feeding.

Benefits of Breast Feeding

After World War II, breast feeding declined dramatically in the United States and most of the Western world. In 1946, 65% of American mothers were breast-feeding their babies. Twenty years later only 27% fed their infants at the breast. By 1983, however, that number shot up again to 61.4%, and the federal government, which advocates infant breast feeding, has set a goal of 75% by 1990.

One reason for this resurgence was the discovery that breast feeding provides both physical and psychological benefits that infant formulas do not. A number of studies, from both developed and developing countries, show that breast-fed babies suffer significantly fewer illnesses, particularly intestinal diseases. Other studies indicate that breast-fed babies suffer less from asthma and are less likely to develop allergies. The reason, scientists have discovered, is that breast milk contains a host of substances that help protect the baby. These materials include a number of immunogens, substances that make antibodies to attack disease-causing organisms. One of these — secretory IgA — produces antibodies against a wide range of bacteria and viruses. Together, the protective substances in breast milk apparently help ward off such ailments as respiratory infections, meningitis (inflammation of the membranes covering the brain and spinal cord), gastroenteritis (inflammation of the mucous membrane that lines the stomach and the intestines), chronic otitis media (inflammation of the middle ear), hay fever, asthma, eczema (itching and scaling skin), and cow's-milk allergy.

Breast feeding also helps the *bonding* of mother and child better than bottle feeding, and aids the infant in developing a sense of trust. With breast feeding, the baby gets the maximum stimulation that comes from a mother's touch and smell, her rhythmic heartbeat, and the taste of her milk. Such stimulation is a factor in a baby's growth and development. Some recent research suggests breast feeding makes for a better relationship between mother and child later in the child's life.

During pregnancy, a woman's body stores 8 to 10 pounds of nutrients to be used to make milk. The hormone prolactin regulates her milk production. This hormone is kept at low levels during pregnancy by the hormones estrogen and progesterone, which are made in the placenta. In the final months of pregnancy, the breasts produce colostrum, or early milk, a yellowish liquid that is the baby's food for the first day or two of life. At birth, the delivery of the placenta triggers production of high levels of prolactin, and with this the flow of breast milk begins.

The breast's milk-secreting cells extract water, lactose (milk sugar), amino acids (the chemical building blocks of proteins), fats, vitamins, minerals, and other substances from

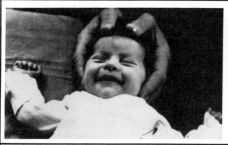 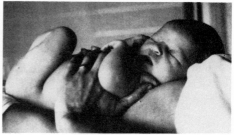

A baby delivered by a drug-free method of childbirth that supporters claim is safer than a medicated labor and delivery.

the mother's blood. The cells convert these nutrients into milk, and then eject the fluid into tiny tubes, called ductules. The milk flows into the lactiferous sinuses, small reservoirs near the nipple, where it is available to the baby on demand.

Drug Concentrations in Breast Milk

If a woman is using a drug, licit or illicit, some of it will almost certainly be extracted from her blood and enter her breast milk. Some drugs are found in equal or higher concentrations in breast milk than in the bloodstream. These include most antihistamines (which are found in many cold and sinus medications and are also used to treat allergies), the group of antibiotics called erythromycins, the antiasthma drug theophylline, and the antituberculosis medication isoniazid. Other drugs are found in lower concentrations in the mother's milk than in her blood. These include barbiturates, diuretics, and penicillin. The presence of a drug in the breast milk reveals nothing about the amount absorbed by the infant, or the drug's effect on the child. Indeed, far less is known about the short- and long-term effects on a child of the mother's drug use during breast feeding than is known about what drugs will enter her milk.

Harmful Medications

Nonetheless, some drugs are known to cause adverse effects for the mother or her breast-fed baby. A woman who resumes taking oral contraceptives may find she produces less milk. Some drugs will interfere with a baby's growth and development. Others may alter the delicate salt and water balance in infants, which can have serious consequences. Antithyroid medications in the mother's milk can damage the baby's thyroid. (Taken during pregnancy, high doses of antithyroid medication can cause mental retardation in the fetus.)

The American Academy of Pediatrics Committee on Drugs has provided physicians with a list of medicines that should not be used during breast feeding. These drugs are:

Bromocriptine (Parlodel), used for several medical problems, including Parkinson's disease, can suppress the secretion of breast milk.

Cimetidine (Tagamet), effective in treating stomach and duodenal (upper part of the small intestine) ulcers, may suppress gastric acid, inhibit drug metabolism, and cause nervousness in the baby.

Clemastine (Tavist), a prescription antihistamine used to treat allergic rhinitis (hay fever), can cause drowsiness, irritability, refusal to feed, a high-pitched cry, and neck stiffness in the infant.

Cyclophosphamide (Cytoxan, Neosar), an anticancer drug, damages an infant's immune system.

Ergotamine (Bellergal, Cafergot, Cafetrate-PB, Ergomar, Ergostat, Gynergen, Medihaler, Wigraine, Wigrettes), used to relieve migraine headaches, may cause vomiting, diarrhea, and convulsions in breast-fed babies.

Gold salts (Myochrysine), used in the treatment of rheumatoid arthritis, may produce a rash and also inflammation of the infant's kidney and liver.

Methotrexate (Mexate) is another anticancer drug that may damage a baby's immune system. Information on the adverse effects of other anticancer drugs is not available.

Phenindione (Hedulin), a medication to prevent blood clots, can cause hemorrhage in the infant.

Other Drugs to Avoid. Other authorities regard additional drugs as unsuitable for use during breast feeding. These include a large number of water pills known as thiazide diuretics, which can suppress the milk supply; cascara sagrada (Aromatic Cascara Fluidextract, others), a prescription laxative that may cause diarrhea in breast-fed babies; and coumarin derivatives (Coumadin, Dicumarol, Panwarfin), anticlotting drugs that lead to bleeding problems in infants. Pharmaceutical companies often recommend against breast feeding while taking certain medications — not because the drugs are *known* to cause problems, but because there are theoretical reasons to suspect they might.

Certain drugs may require the mother to stop breast-feeding for a time. Metronidazole (Flagyl) is an anti-infective drug most often used to treat genital and urinary tract infections. It has been found to cause cancer in mice and rats. The American Academy of Pediatrics (AAP) recommends that mothers discontinue breast-feeding for 12 to 24 hours after taking the medicine so that the substance can be excreted from their bodies. The other entries on the AAP's list of drugs that require a temporary halt to breast feeding are all radioactive chemicals used for various diagnostic studies. These include gallium 69 (present in breast milk for two weeks), iodine 125 (present for 12 days), iodine 131 (present for 2 to 14 days, depending on the type of study), radioactive sodium (present for 96 hours) and three forms of technetium 99m (present 15 to 72 hours).

Illicit Drugs and their Dangers

Illicit drugs also pass into breast milk. Doctors have long known that an opiate-addicted mother who breast feeds can cause her child to become addicted too. Moreover, the babies of narcotic-addicted women tend to have a significantly poorer sucking rate and thus take in fewer nutrients per feeding. Narcotics taken medically as painkillers are given in small enough doses that they are unlikely to cause a nursing baby any problems.

Significant quantities of the most psychoactive ingredient in marijuana enter the breast milk of pot-smoking mothers and the blood of their nursing infants. Animal studies show marijuana exposure reduces the mother's milk production, probably because the drug impairs the secretion of prolactin. The effect in humans is less clear. But in its comprehensive report on marijuana, the National Academy of Sciences' Institute of Medicine warned that marijuana "can be secreted in breast milk and therefore, can be toxic" to nursing babies.

PCP also enters breast milk. Little is known about its effects on babies through breast feeding. But given its terrible results in adults and the newborns of PCP users, the chances are great that it can cause serious problems in nursing infants.

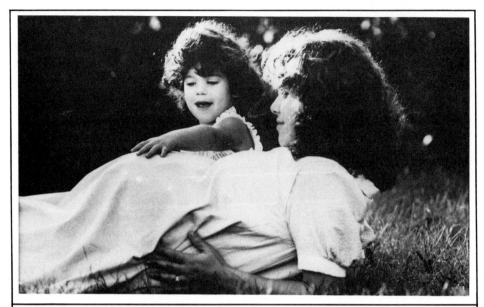

A healthy toddler and her mother enjoy a quiet moment. Women who get adequate prenatal care and exercise caution concerning the use of drugs during pregnancy help assure the health of their children.

Nonprescription drugs and other chemicals consumed by a woman can also reach her baby through breast milk. Regular, high doses of aspirin, for example, may cause a tendency to bleed easily in an infant. There is evidence that over-the-counter antihistamines may decrease milk production, and concern that in high doses they may cause excitement, hallucinations, or even convulsions in the baby.

Nicotine passes into breast milk, and the more a mother smokes, the more nicotine reaches her child. Moderate cigarette smoking does not appear to cause problems. But several breast-fed children whose mothers were very heavy smokers have suffered nicotine poisoning. Some evidence suggests that nicotine may reduce the secretion of breast milk. If a woman feels she must smoke, she should do it immediately after breast-feeding her baby, and then refrain from smoking until after the next feeding.

Alcohol also can reduce the quantity of milk available to the baby. It can cause drowsiness in an infant, and if the mother drinks heavily before nursing, the child, too, may become drunk. Caffeine passes into breast milk, but there are conflicting reports about its effects. Some doctors believe that heavy consumption of caffeine by the mother can cause agitation in the nursing child. They suggest breast-feeding women cut down on coffee, tea, and soft drinks containing caffeine.

Of course, a glass of wine, or a morning cup of coffee, or even certain medications are not incompatible with breast feeding. Basically, the same advice applies in breast feeding as in pregnancy.

1. Avoid using illicit drugs.
2. Do not take unneeded or unprescribed medications.
3. Finally, do not refuse to take a recommended drug without first discussing this decision with your doctor.

APPENDIX

State Agencies
for the Prevention and Treatment
of Drug Abuse

ALABAMA
Department of Mental Health
Division of Mental Illness and
 Substance Abuse Community
 Programs
200 Interstate Park Drive
P.O. Box 3710
Montgomery, AL 36193
(205) 271-9253

ALASKA
Department of Health and Social
 Services
Office of Alcoholism and Drug
 Abuse
Pouch H-05-F
Juneau, AK 99811
(907) 586-6201

ARIZONA
Department of Health Services
Division of Behavioral Health
 Services
Bureau of Community Services
Alcohol Abuse and Alcoholism
 Section
2500 East Van Buren
Phoenix, AZ 85008
(602) 255-1238

Department of Health Services
Division of Behavioral Health
 Services
Bureau of Community Services
Drug Abuse Section
2500 East Van Buren
Phoenix, AZ 85008
(602) 255-1240

ARKANSAS
Department of Human Services
Office on Alcohol and Drug Abuse
 Prevention
1515 West 7th Avenue
Suite 310
Little Rock, AR 72202
(501) 371-2603

CALIFORNIA
Department of Alcohol and Drug
 Abuse
111 Capitol Mall
Sacramento, CA 95814
(916) 445-1940

COLORADO
Department of Health
Alcohol and Drug Abuse Division
4210 East 11th Avenue
Denver, CO 80220
(303) 320-6137

CONNECTICUT
Alcohol and Drug Abuse
 Commission
999 Asylum Avenue
3rd Floor
Hartford, CT 06105
(203) 566-4145

DELAWARE
Division of Mental Health
Bureau of Alcoholism and Drug
 Abuse
1901 North Dupont Highway
Newcastle, DE 19720
(302) 421-6101

DISTRICT OF COLUMBIA
Department of Human Services
Office of Health Planning and
   Development
601 Indiana Avenue, NW
Suite 500
Washington, D.C. 20004
(202) 724-5641

FLORIDA
Department of Health and
   Rehabilitative Services
Alcoholic Rehabilitation Program
1317 Winewood Boulevard
Room 187A
Tallahassee, FL 32301
(904) 488-0396

Department of Health and
   Rehabilitative Services
Drug Abuse Program
1317 Winewood Boulevard
Building 6, Room 155
Tallahassee, FL 32301
(904) 488-0900

GEORGIA
Department of Human Resources
Division of Mental Health and
   Mental Retardation
Alcohol and Drug Section
618 Ponce De Leon Avenue, NE
Atlanta, GA 30365-2101
(404) 894-4785

HAWAII
Department of Health
Mental Health Division
Alcohol and Drug Abuse Branch
1250 Punch Bowl Street
P.O. Box 3378
Honolulu, HI 96801
(808) 548-4280

IDAHO
Department of Health and Welfare
Bureau of Preventive Medicine
Substance Abuse Section
450 West State
Boise, ID 83720
(208) 334-4368

ILLINOIS
Department of Mental Health and
   Developmental Disabilities
Division of Alcoholism
160 North La Salle Street
Room 1500
Chicago, IL 60601
(312) 793-2907

Illinois Dangerous Drugs
   Commission
300 North State Street
Suite 1500
Chicago, IL 60610
(312) 822-9860

INDIANA
Department of Mental Health
Division of Addiction Services
429 North Pennsylvania Street
Indianapolis, IN 46204
(317) 232-7816

IOWA
Department of Substance Abuse
505 5th Avenue
Insurance Exchange Building
Suite 202
Des Moines, IA 50319
(515) 281-3641

KANSAS
Department of Social Rehabilitation
Alcohol and Drug Abuse Services
2700 West 6th Street
Biddle Building
Topeka, KS 66606
(913) 296-3925

KENTUCKY
Cabinet for Human Resources
Department of Health Services
Substance Abuse Branch
275 East Main Street
Frankfort, KY 40601
(502) 564-2880

LOUISIANA
Department of Health and Human
  Resources
Office of Mental Health and
  Substance Abuse
655 North 5th Street
P.O. Box 4049
Baton Rouge, LA 70821
(504) 342-2565

MAINE
Department of Human Services
Office of Alcoholism and Drug
  Abuse Prevention
Bureau of Rehabilitation
32 Winthrop Street
Augusta, ME 04330
(207) 289-2781

MARYLAND
Alcoholism Control Administration
201 West Preston Street
Fourth Floor
Baltimore, MD 21201
(301) 383-2977

State Health Department
Drug Abuse Administration
201 West Preston Street
Baltimore, MD 21201
(301) 383-3312

MASSACHUSETTS
Department of Public Health
Division of Alcoholism
755 Boylston Street
Sixth Floor
Boston, MA 02116
(617) 727-1960

Department of Public Health
Division of Drug Rehabilitation
600 Washington Street
Boston, MA 02114
(617) 727-8617

MICHIGAN
Department of Public Health
Office of Substance Abuse Services
3500 North Logan Street
P.O. Box 30035
Lansing, MI 48909
(517) 373-8603

MINNESOTA
Department of Public Welfare
Chemical Dependency Program
  Division
Centennial Building
658 Cedar Street
4th Floor
Saint Paul, MN 55155
(612) 296-4614

MISSISSIPPI
Department of Mental Health
Division of Alcohol and Drug Abuse
1102 Robert E. Lee Building
Jackson, MS 39201
(601) 359-1297

MISSOURI
Department of Mental Health
Division of Alcoholism and Drug
  Abuse
2002 Missouri Boulevard
P.O. Box 687
Jefferson City, MO 65102
(314) 751-4942

MONTANA
Department of Institutions
Alcohol and Drug Abuse Division
1539 11th Avenue
Helena, MT 59620
(406) 449-2827

NEBRASKA
Department of Public Institutions
Division of Alcoholism and Drug Abuse
801 West Van Dorn Street
P.O. Box 94728
Lincoln, NB 68509
(402) 471-2851, Ext. 415

NEVADA
Department of Human Resources
Bureau of Alcohol and Drug Abuse
505 East King Street
Carson City, NV 89710
(702) 885-4790

NEW HAMPSHIRE
Department of Health and Welfare
Office of Alcohol and Drug Abuse
 Prevention
Hazen Drive
Health and Welfare Building
Concord, NH 03301
(603) 271-4627

NEW JERSEY
Department of Health
Division of Alcoholism
129 East Hanover Street CN 362
Trenton, NJ 08625
(609) 292-8949

Department of Health
Division of Narcotic and Drug Abuse
 Control
129 East Hanover Street CN 362
Trenton, NJ 08625
(609) 292-8949

NEW MEXICO
Health and Environment Department
Behavioral Services Division
Substance Abuse Bureau
725 Saint Michaels Drive
P.O. Box 968
Santa Fe, NM 87503
(505) 984-0020, Ext. 304

NEW YORK
Division of Alcoholism and Alcohol
 Abuse
194 Washington Avenue
Albany, NY 12210
(518) 474-5417

Division of Substance Abuse
 Services
Executive Park South
Box 8200
Albany, NY 12203
(518) 457-7629

NORTH CAROLINA
Department of Human Resources
Division of Mental Health, Mental
 Retardation and Substance Abuse
 Services
Alcohol and Drug Abuse Services
325 North Salisbury Street
Albemarle Building
Raleigh, NC 27611
(919) 733-4670

NORTH DAKOTA
Department of Human Services
Division of Alcoholism and Drug
 Abuse
State Capitol Building
Bismarck, ND 58505
(701) 224-2767

OHIO
Department of Health
Division of Alcoholism
246 North High Street
P.O. Box 118
Columbus, OH 43216
(614) 466-3543

Department of Mental Health
Bureau of Drug Abuse
65 South Front Street
Columbus, OH 43215
(614) 466-9023

OKLAHOMA
Department of Mental Health
Alcohol and Drug Programs
4545 North Lincoln Boulevard
Suite 100 East Terrace
P.O. Box 53277
Oklahoma City, OK 73152
(405) 521-0044

OREGON
Department of Human Resources
Mental Health Division
Office of Programs for Alcohol and
    Drug Problems
2575 Bittern Street, NE
Salem, OR 97310
(503) 378-2163

PENNSYLVANIA
Department of Health
Office of Drug and Alcohol
    Programs
Commonwealth and Forster Avenues
Health and Welfare Building
P.O. Box 90
Harrisburg, PA 17108
(717) 787-9857

RHODE ISLAND
Department of Mental Health,
    Mental Retardation and Hospitals
Division of Substance Abuse
Substance Abuse Administration
    Building
Cranston, RI 02920
(401) 464-2091

SOUTH CAROLINA
Commission on Alcohol and Drug
    Abuse
3700 Forest Drive
Columbia, SC 29204
(803) 758-2521

SOUTH DAKOTA
Department of Health
Division of Alcohol and Drug Abuse
523 East Capitol, Joe Foss Building
Pierre, SD 57501
(605) 773-4806

TENNESSEE
Department of Mental Health and
    Mental Retardation
Alcohol and Drug Abuse Services
505 Deaderick Street
James K. Polk Building, Fourth Floor
Nashville, TN 37219
(615) 741-1921

TEXAS
Commission on Alcoholism
809 Sam Houston State Office Building
Austin, TX 78701
(512) 475-2577

Department of Community Affairs
Drug Abuse Prevention Division
2015 South Interstate Highway 35
P.O. Box 13166
Austin, TX 78711
(512) 443-4100

UTAH
Department of Social Services
Division of Alcoholism and Drugs
150 West North Temple
Suite 350
P.O. Box 2500
Salt Lake City, UT 84110
(801) 533-6532

VERMONT
Agency of Human Services
Department of Social and
    Rehabilitation Services
Alcohol and Drug Abuse Division
103 South Main Street
Waterbury, VT 05676
(802) 241-2170

VIRGINIA
Department of Mental Health and
   Mental Retardation
Division of Substance Abuse
109 Governor Street
P.O. Box 1797
Richmond, VA 23214
(804) 786-5313

WASHINGTON
Department of Social and Health
   Service
Bureau of Alcohol and Substance
   Abuse
Office Building—44 W
Olympia, WA 98504
(206) 753-5866

WEST VIRGINIA
Department of Health
Office of Behavioral Health Services
Division on Alcoholism and Drug
   Abuse
1800 Washington Street East
Building 3 Room 451
Charleston, WV 25305
(304) 348-2276

WISCONSIN
Department of Health and Social
   Services
Division of Community Services
Bureau of Community Programs
Alcohol and Other Drug Abuse
   Program Office
1 West Wilson Street
P.O. Box 7851
Madison, WI 53707
(608) 266-2717

WYOMING
Alcohol and Drug Abuse Programs
Hathaway Building
Cheyenne, WY 82002
(307) 777-7115, Ext. 7118

GUAM
Mental Health & Substance Abuse
   Agency
P.O. Box 20999
Guam 96921

PUERTO RICO
Department of Addiction Control
   Services
Alcohol Abuse Programs
P.O. Box B-Y Rio Piedras Station
Rio Piedras, PR 00928
(809) 763-5014

Department of Addiction Control
   Services
Drug Abuse Programs
P.O. Box B-Y Rio Piedras Station
Rio Piedras, PR 00928
(809) 764-8140

VIRGIN ISLANDS
Division of Mental Health,
   Alcoholism & Drug Dependency
   Services
P.O. Box 7329
Saint Thomas, Virgin Islands 00801
(809) 774-7265

AMERICAN SAMOA
LBJ Tropical Medical Center
Department of Mental Health Clinic
Pago Pago, American Samoa 96799

TRUST TERRITORIES
Director of Health Services
Office of the High Commissioner
Saipan, Trust Territories 96950

Further Reading

Feldman, George B., M.D., with Felshman, Anne. *The Complete Handbook of Pregnancy*. New York: G.P. Putnam's Sons, 1984.

Golbus, Mitchell S., M.D. "Teratology for the Obstetrician: Current Status." *Journal of the American College of Obstetricians and Gynecologists*, March 1980.

Goldberg, Larry H., M.D., and Leahy, Joann, M.D. *The Doctors' Guide to Medication During Pregnancy and Lactation*. New York: Quill, 1984.

Heinonen, Olli P., M.D., M.Sc.; Slone, Dennis, M.D.; and Shapiro, Samuel, F.R.C.P. *Birth Defects and Drugs in Pregnancy*. Littleton, MA: Publishing Sciences Group, 1977.

Holt, Linda Hughey, M.D., and Weber, Melva. *Book of WomanCare*. New York: Random House, 1981, 1982.

Kitzinger, Sheila. *The Complete Book of Pregnancy and Childbirth*. New York: Alfred A. Knopf, 1985.

Parish, Peter, M.D. *The Doctors and Patients Handbook of Medicines and Drugs*. New York: Alfred A. Knopf, 1977.

Glossary

abruptio placentae: premature separation of the placenta from the uterus wall

acetaminophen: a nonaspirin, nonprescription pain reliever

amniotic fluid: fluid inside the amniotic sac. It is 98% or more water and contains body salts, carbohydrates, fats, enzymes, hormones, and pigments

amniotic sac: fluid-filled membrane surrounding the fetus. Also called the amnion

antihypertensives: drugs used to lower high blood pressure

Apgar system: rating system that judges the health of newborns

biotransformation: the body's process of altering a drug for excretion by changing its chemical structure. Also called drug breakdown or drug metabolism

Brazelton scale: series of 27 reaction tests used to assess the behavior of newborns

caffeine: a mild stimulant that is found in some foods, beverages, and nonprescription drugs

carbon dioxide: waste gas that results when cells "burn" oxygen for energy

carbon monoxide: colorless, odorless gas that kills in large doses. The gas enters the bloodstream when cigarette smoke is inhaled; it reduces the amount of oxygen carried by red blood cells

chromosomes: structures within the cells that contain the genes

cocaine: illicit, psychologically addictive drug from the coca plant; creates euphoria, feelings of energy and confidence

Collaborative Perinatal Project: federal government study of over 50,000 pregnancies that kept data on the children up to age 7

colostrum: early milk; infant's first food from the breast

convulsion: sudden, violent, uncontrolled muscle spasm; sometimes accompanied by unconsciousness

deoxyribonucleic acid: DNA; the material from which genes are made

drug: substance that changes the structure or functioning of a living organism

embryo: the developing organism during the early stages of life in the womb; in humans the embryonic stage occurs between two and eight weeks after fertilization of egg

enzymes: substances produced by cells that start or accelerate specific chemical reactions such as the breakdown of drugs in the body

epilepsy: disorder involving the brain's nerve cells; causes sudden loss of consciousness, sometimes convulsions

estrogens: group of female sex hormones made mostly in the ovaries. They help regulate reproductive functions and maintain female secondary sex characteristics

ethanol: specific form of alcohol in beer, wine, and distilled spirits

fallopian tubes: the two tubes through which eggs travel when passing from the ovaries to the uterus

fat-soluble drugs: drugs easily dissolved in fat; must be converted to water-soluble drugs before the body can excrete them

fetal alcohol effects: term that describes alcohol-caused birth defects less serious than those of full fetal alcohol syndrome

fetal alcohol syndrome: specific set of physical and mental handicaps caused by a mother's heavy drinking during pregnancy. These include growth deficiency, a particular pattern of facial deformities, brain and spinal cord defects, and varying degrees of malformations in major organs

fetus: the developing organism during the later stages of life in the womb; in humans the fetal stage occurs from eight weeks after fertilization of the egg until birth

genes: materials inside each cell that carry the directions the body uses to make the various proteins it needs. Genes determine such things as eye and hair color and susceptibility to certain diseases

hallucination: a sensory impression that has no basis in reality

hallucinogen: a drug that induces hallucinations

heroin: an opiate; not used medically in the United States; heroin is physically addictive and a major drug of abuse

hyperactivity: disruptive pattern of behavior that includes excitability, overactivity, poor concentration, and short attention span

lysergic acid diethylamide (LSD): psychoactive drug that changes a user's perceptions of time, distance, color, and form. LSD can cause acute, terrifying panic and psychiatric problems

marijuana: dried leaves and flowers of *cannabis sativa*, or hemp plant. A psychoactive drug that produces mild euphoria and hallucinations

metabolites: chemical products that result when enzymes in the body break down drugs

methadone: a synthetic narcotic used to treat heroin addicts

miscarriage: death and natural expulsion of a fetus

morphine: an opiate used in medicine as a painkiller; is also physically addictive

nicotine: poisonous chemical contained in cigarette smoke; causes blood vessels, including those in the placenta, to narrow and reduce the flow of oxygen to the fetus

opiates: opium and other narcotic drugs derived from it

opium: powerful narcotic produced from the juice of the opium poppy

ovaries: two female glands — one on each side of the uterus — that produce eggs and female sex hormones

perinatal: period shortly before, during, and soon after birth

phencyclidine (PCP): illicit drug; can cause mental confusion, hallucinations, muscle rigidity, seizures, violent behavior. Also known as "angel dust"

placenta: organ that allows life-sustaining oxygen and nutrients to pass from a pregnant woman to her fetus, and through which wastes from the fetus pass to be excreted by the mother

placental membrane: thin membrane of fetal tissue that physically separates the mother's blood from that of her fetus. Oxygen, nutrients, and other substances in the mother's blood must pass through it to reach the fetus

progesterone: female sex hormone responsible for preparing the uterus to receive the fertilized egg

prolactin: hormone that stimulates breast-milk production

psychoactive drugs: chemicals that alter the functioning of the brain and that may cause such things as euphoria, hallucinations, and psychiatric disorders

side effect: an unwanted and unintentional reaction to a drug

sudden infant death syndrome (SIDS): sudden, unexpected death of an apparently healthy baby for which no cause can be found. Usually occurs between one and six months of age

teratogen: any substance taken during pregnancy that can cause a physical, mental, or behavioral defect in a child

thalidomide: a drug, once prescribed for treating morning sickness in pregnant women, that caused severe birth defects

uterus: female organ in which an unborn child develops and is nourished

water-soluble drugs: drugs easily dissolved in water. They are removed unchanged from the blood for excretion by the body, mostly in the urine

Picture Credits

American Cancer Society: p. 52; AP/Wide World Photos: pp. 11, 22, 32, 35, 42, 55, 65, 71, 74, 91; Art Resource: pp. 18, 84; The Bettmann Archive: pp. 9, 20, 46, 65, 83; Frank DeRosa, R.Ph., courtesy of: p. 38; Food and Drug Administration: p. 79; March of Dimes Birth Defect Foundation: p. 59; National Institute of Health Library: p. 60; New York Department of Health: p. 49; David N. Phillips/ The Population Council: p. 30; Press Telegram/Bob Amaral: p. 70; UPI/Bettmann Newsphotos: pp. 13, 50, 62, 72, 76, 87; Washington Post (Reprinted by permission of D. C. Public Library): p. 68.

Gary Tong (original illustrations): pp. 25, 28, 36, 40

Index

abruptio placentae, 57, 68
Accutane *see* isotretinoin
acetaldehyde, 48
acetaminophen (Datril; Excedrin;
    Tylenol), 34, 82
alcohol, 43–44, 63, 82
    breast feeding and, 90–91
    fetal development and, 21, 23, 31,
        37, 45–48
    metabolism, 48
    pregnancy and, 50–51, 54
    see also fetal alcohol syndrome;
        pregnancy
alcoholism, 43–45
American Academy of Pediatrics, 76, 88,
    89
aminopterin, 78
amnion *see* amniotic sac
amniotic fluid, 36–37, 48
amniotic sac, 26, 36
amphetamines, 70–73
androgens, 78
angel dust *see* phencyclidine
anticancer drugs, 78
anticoagulants, 77–78
anticonvulsants, 75, 76, 77
antihistamines, 87, 88, 90
antithyroid drugs, 80–81, 88
Apgar score, 58
aspirin, 82, 90

barbiturates, 73, 87
bilirubin, 28
birth defects, 31
    causes, 37–39
    factors affecting, 39–40, 47–49, 76
    see also fetus; pregnancy
birth weight, 54–56, 67, 80, 81
    see also smoking
bonding, 86
Book of WomanCare (Holt and Weber),
    83
Brazelton scale, 69
breast feeding, 85–87
    drug use and, 21, 87–91
bromocriptine (Parlodel), 88

cadmium, 31, 37, 59
    see also smoking
caffeine, 82–83, 91
carbon monoxide, 60–61
carboxyhemoglobin, 61
cascara sagrada, 88
cataracts, 79
cell division, 24–25
cellular growth factors, 27
central nervous system depressants, 44
chloroquine (Aralen), 81
chromosomes, 24, 67
cigarette smoke, 59–61
    see also smoking
cimetidine (Tagamet), 88
cirrhosis, 44
    see also alcohol
clemastine (Tavist), 88
clomiphene citrate (Clomid; Serophene),
    78
cocaine, 68–69
codeine, 64
Collaborative Perinatal Project, 58, 78
colostrum, 86
coumarin, 88
crashing, 71
cretinism, 80
cyanide, 60
cyclophosphamide (Cytoxan; Neosar), 88

delta-9-tetrahydrocannibinol, 66
deoxyribonucleic acid (DNA), 39
dependence, 44
DES *see* diethylstilbestrol
diethylstilbestrol (DES), 37, 41, 78
    see also birth defects
dihydrotachysterol, 81
diuretics, 75, 87, 88
DNA *see* deoxyribonucleic acid
drugs
    biotransformation, 33–36
    definition, 33
    fat-soluble, 34, 35
    fetal development and, 31, 34–39
    interactions, 34–35, 49
    medical uses, 33

metabolites, 30–31, 34–38, 48
over-the-counter, 81–82
water-soluble, 33–35

egg, 24
embryo, development, 24–26, 39
    see also fetus, development
enzymes, 34
ergotamine (Bellergal; Cafergot; Cafetrate-
    PB), 88
erythromycin, 87
estrogens, 27, 41, 78
ethanol, 44
    see also alcohol
ethyl alcohol *see* alcohol

FAE *see* fetal alcohol effects
fallopian tube, 24–25, 41
FAS *see* fetal alcohol syndrome
fertilization, 24–25
fertilization membrane, 24
fetal alcohol effects (FAE), 47–48
fetal alcohol syndrome (FAS), 21, 43–49
fetal hydantoin syndrome, 77
fetus
    alcohol and, 47–49
    blood supply, 27–30, 37, 40
    development, 25–26, 40–41
    genetic makeup, 24, 39
    heavy metals and, 31
    narcotic addiction, 64–66
    nourishment of, 27–29, 37, 60–61
    smoking and, 49, 59–61
    viruses and, 29
    see also birth defects; pregnancy
folic acid antagonists, 78
Food and Drug Administration, U.S., 79,
    82, 83

gastroenteritis, 86
gold salts (Myochrysine), 88

Harvey, William, 27
heparin (Lipo-Hepin), 78
hepatitis, 44
heroin, 64–66
Hippocrates, 64
hormones, 41
hydrocephaly, 77
hyperkinesis, 58
hyperthyroidism, 80
hypothyroidism, 80

immunogens, 86
Institute of Medicine (National Academy
    of Sciences), 54, 67, 90
intrauterine growth retardation (IUGR),
    56
iodides, 80
isoniazid, 87
isotretinoin (Accutane), 37, 77
IUGR *see* intrauterine growth retardation

lactiferous sinuses, 87
lead, 31, 59–60
lithium (Eskalith; Lithane), 80
LSD *see* lysergic acid diethylamide
lysergic acid diethylamide (LSD), 73

manic-depressives, 80
marijuana, 20, 63, 66–68, 89
meningitis, 86
mental retardation, 46, 48, 80, 88
meperidine (Demerol; Mepergan), 64
methadone, 64–66
methimazole, 80
methotrexate (Mexate), 78, 88
metronidazole (Flagyl), 89
morphine, 64–65

narcolepsy, 71
National Institute on Alcohol Abuse and
    Alcoholism, 45
nicotine, 60–61, 90

opiates, 64–66
oral contraceptives, 78–79, 87
otitis media, 86
ovaries, 24
ovum *see* egg

Parkinson's disease, 88
passive immunity, 29
PCP *see* phencyclidine
pentazocine (Talwin), 64
phencyclidine (PCP), 63, 69–70, 89
phenindione (Hedulin), 88
phenytoin (Dilantin), 77
placenta, 20, 26–27, 35–36, 40, 57,
    59–60, 68, 82, 86
    barrier function, 27, 29–30
    see also fetus; pregnancy
placenta previa, 57
placental barrier, 30
placental membrane, 27–28

pregnancy
  alcohol and, 43–51
  amphetamines and, 70–73
  barbiturates and, 73
  caffeine and, 82–83
  cocaine and, 68–69
  drug metabolism and, 35–37
  ectopic, 41
  guidelines for drug use during, 38,
    50–51, 75–76, 83
  LSD and, 73
  marijuana and, 66–68
  medications and, 31, 37, 75–82
  opiates and, 64–66
  phencyclidine and, 70
  smoking and, 53–61
  see also birth defects; drugs; fetus
progesterone, 27, 78
prolactin, 86
propranolol (Inderal), 81
propylthiouracil (Propacil), 80
protein hormones, 27

radioisotopes, 81, 89–90
rejection mechanism, 26
rubella virus, 39

scoliosis, 43
secretory IgA, 86
SIDS see sudden infant death syndrome
smoking
  birth defects and, 58–59
  birth weight and, 54–56, 59–61
  breast feeding and, 90
  complications of pregnancy due to,
    56–57

epidemiology of, 53–54
fetal development and, 21, 23, 31, 49
health risks, 53
health warnings, 53
respiratory illnesses due to, 57–58
see also pregnancy
sperm, 24
steroid hormones, 27
streptomycin, 79
sudden infant death syndrome (SIDS),
  56–57, 69
  see also smoking
Surgeon General, U.S., 51, 53, 54
syphilis, 29, 37

teratogens, 37–39, 44, 66
tetracycline (Achromycin; Robitet), 37,
  79
thalidomide, 31, 34, 38, 40, 75
theophylline, 87
thiocyanate, 60
tobacco see smoking
tolerance, 44, 47
trimethadione (Tridione), 77

umbilical cord, 28–29
urea, 28
uric acid, 28
uterus, 24–26

warfarin (Coumadin; Panwarfin), 78
Wharton's jelly, 28

yolk sac, 26

Patrick Young is a science and medical correspondent for the Newhouse News Service in Washington, D.C. In 1979, he served on the senior staff of the Presidential Commission that investigated the nuclear power plant accident at Three Mile Island. He is the author of *Asthma and Allergies: An Optimistic Future* and *Drifting Continents, Shifting Seas: An Introduction to Plate Tectonics,* a book for young adults. He has been honored with over a dozen awards for his articles on medicine, the physical sciences, psychology, and space.

Solomon H. Snyder, M.D., is Distinguished Service Professor of Neuroscience, Pharmacology and Psychiatry at The Johns Hopkins University School of Medicine. He has served as president of the Society for Neuroscience and in 1978 received the Albert Lasker Award in Medical Research. He has authored *Uses of Marijuana, Madness and the Brain, The Troubled Mind, Biological Aspects of Mental Disorder,* and edited *Perspective in Neuropharmacology: A Tribute to Julius Axelrod.* Professor Snyder was a research associate with Dr. Axelrod at the National Institutes of Health.

Barry L. Jacobs, Ph.D., is currently a professor in the program of neuroscience at Princeton University. Professor Jacobs is author of *Serotonin Neurotransmission and Behavior* and *Hallucinogens: Neurochemical, Behavioral and Clinical Perspectives.* He has written many journal articles in the field of neuroscience and contributed numerous chapters to books on behavior and brain science. He has been a member of several panels of the National Institute of Mental Health.

Joann Ellison Rodgers, M.S. (Columbia), became Deputy Director of Public Affairs and Director of Media Relations for the Johns Hopkins Medical Institutions in Baltimore, Maryland, in 1984 after 18 years as an award-winning science journalist and widely read columnist for the Hearst newspapers.

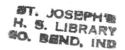